How to Succeed on...

Keto

Without Really

Trying

Nissa Graun

From

Eating Fat is the New Skinny

Dedication:

So, I guess I have to dedicate this book to my husband Jason...but not for all of the mushy, gushy reasons wives typically dedicate books to their husbands. For now, let's just say I'm dedicating this book to my husband because - poop sticks. You'll completely understand once you get to chapter 7.

If you are reading the paperback version of this book, I've added a complete link library at the end of the book in the event you'd like more info during your journey.

How to Succeed on Keto Without Really Trying Keto With Results!

Table of Contents

No table of contents entries found.

Nissa Graun
Before: 245 lbs   After: 135 lbs

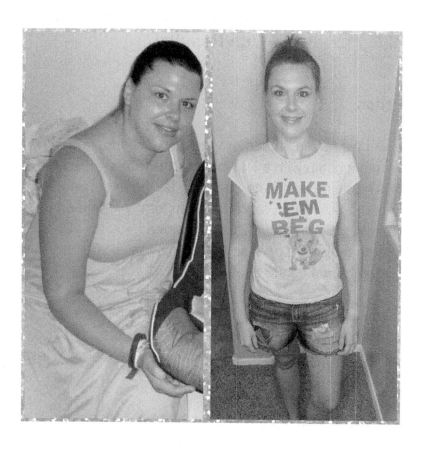

How to Succeed on Keto Without Really Trying Keto With Results!

Introduction

In the event we haven't made proper introductions, I want to start our relationship with a little more transparency than the title of this book implies. Keto seems to be the latest and greatest diet buzzword. Everywhere you turn, you find another amazing keto success story. Every newsfeed you scroll, there's another Jen, Jill or Jane that wants to sell you her magic potion to make keto easy for you!

The truth is … keto ain't easy! If drastically slashing carbs while substantially raising fat every single day was as easy as others make it sound, everyone would simply cut carbs to less than 20 and drop body fat like it's hot!

"If yo' keto expert cop a attitude, drop him like he's hot, drop him like he's hot, drop him like he's hot."

Sorry, I've been at OrangeTheory Fitness a lot lately, and sometimes I just break into song completely out of nowhere. Thanks Snoop Dog for your contribution to keep my workouts at max force. Seriously - ketones, a fasted workout and Snoop Dog - that's some keto magic right there.

As you'll learn throughout this book, I veer off on pop culture related tangents quite often. You'll also learn I attempted keto type diets for years and failed miserably, low carb diet after low carb diet. I never realized I was failing miserably at the time. I saw the number on the scale move down, often rather quickly, so I always counted my low carb attempts as a success.

While I'd always lose weight with each low carb attempt, I'd also always gain all of the weight back within a few months. Being in a constant cycle of weight loss, followed by weight regain isn't what I'd consider a successful keto plan.

Let me also get back to my gangsta keto rap from above. We'll be chit chatting more about all of the "keto experts" who insist there can only be one way. Basically, if something worked well for them, or a few of their clients, it must work well for everyone else. While I get much more into this throughout the book since this attitude drives me absolutely insane, let's repeat this mantra for now:

"If his keto conviction is too strong, he's probably wrong!"

If you say it in the same tone as Johnny Cochran when presenting the glove at the OJ trial, you're more likely to remember this mantra. This mantra will be important when you bump into those in the keto crowd that have nothing else to do with their day than argue you into submission.

Just as we all know OJ has guilty written all over his extra large running back hands, no matter how tampered the evidence, the experts who claim the same keto approach will work for every single person who tries it are also guilty. They're all guilty of doling out awful advice to innocent keto bystanders. Also, a lot of them are mean.

Why Listen to Me?

So what makes me any better than these know-it-alls on the keto message boards? Who am I to write an entire book about a diet I failed miserably each time I tried it for nearly 20 years?

In case you haven't watched the news lately, I'm that girl who was featured as the nightly teaser for several news stations across the country. I believe one headline used was, "Mom drops 105 pounds by eating fat." Our local station even teased the story with a quote from my interview where I proclaimed in jest, "Half of my diet consists of dark chocolate."

Yep, all of the above is correct. I lost more than 100 pounds with a high fat diet, and a hefty percentage of what I eat consists of dark chocolate in some form. The incorrect part is none of this is a recent news story. All of the hoopla surrounding my shocking truth happened a few years ago.

I was featured in *People Magazine's* 100 pounds down issue in June 2018. Several news outlets throughout the country picked up my story to show their viewers how they too can eat fat and get healthy. Sure, the next week most of these stations probably aired a story about all of the fictional ways a keto diet can kill you, but tomayto, tomahto. At least a little bit of truth was leaked.

I'm not just trying to convince you I'm some kind of hero for making an appearance in a few news stories throughout the country; I do have an actual point. I spoke of my moment in the spotlight to point out - here I am more than two years later, and I'm still living my best keto life. In fact, I made it to my goal weight over three years ago, and I haven't looked back. At least not on the scale.

I finally found information that helped me cheat on a low carb plan, which finally made a low carb lifestyle easy. I never thought I'd have the ability to do things like sit next to a box of open donuts all day long without even a little temptation.

If you were to tell me I also skipped breakfast that day, and there were still no desperate cries in my head for at least one little taste, I'd point and laugh because that's insane. But this scenario actually happened. This is the day I finally knew I arrived!

I spent the previous year putting work in on the less glamorous stuff like improving digestion, ditching all of my processed carb favorites, and dropping fat like it was hot; body fat, not nutritional fat.

My nutritional fat intake skyrocketed, which helped take my keto success to a whole new level.

Since I lost somewhere between 80-90 pounds in a little over a year, I'm sure to outsiders I made this low carb stuff look easy. Now that I'm well past the finish line and I've been hanging out on the sidelines cheering on others for a while, it almost feels like it was way too easy; especially since I went on to lose another 65 pounds after my second pregnancy like it ain't no thang.

Keto Isn't the Quick Fix It's Made Out To Be

I don't want you to think what you're about to read is some quick fix plan that's the miracle you've been praying for. It's not. In fact, that plan doesn't exist. If someone tells you a plan like that exists, run swiftly in the opposite direction.

If you were to find a magical plan that helped you drop weight like hotcakes, I fear the repercussions a plan like that will have on your body long term.

Quick weight loss over a short period of time isn't healthy. I don't even care if a doctor surgically sews up your stomach; most people should never lose more than 1-2 pounds most weeks. Unhealthy weight loss methods will always catch up with you in the end.

I'm not saying you're wrong if you had a surgery like this; I'm just saying I've seen a lot of people still searching for answers once this solution no longer works for them. Slow and steady wins the keto race. (This slow and steady approach also helps keep loose skin in check - bonus!)

I know that's not what you want to hear. After all, keto is this magical plan where everyone who goes on keto drops at least 5 pounds each week, right? Everyone you know that's on keto is having mad success on the plan. Who am I to tell you that keto isn't magical, and you won't drop the 50 pounds it took you years to gain in only a few weeks?

Well, I'm someone that wants to be upfront and honest with you that while forming a ketogenic lifestyle takes hard work, the outcome is so worth the effort you put in. And I'm not just talking weight loss benefits here. There are so many health benefits that can come with eating a well formulated, real food diet that is also low in carbs. (That's a fancy way of saying keto, in case you haven't caught on yet.)

I also want you to learn how to keto the right way, right from the start. If you're in, be in!

Quit following the flashy new diet trend, even if that flashy new trend is just another keto expert telling you it's his way or the highway. You have to figure out the right keto plan that will work with your body chemistry and preferred lifestyle.

I'm not saying you have to follow the same exact path I followed 100% ... but I do want you to know there are a lot of opposing views in the keto community. While some of those views may help you see some progress at the beginning, eventually you'll end up in the land of Weightloss Stalls. That's a land none of us want to visit.

An even worse place to end up is Weight Regainsville. If you go by some of the popular keto advice where many ketoers end up clashing well established Weight Watchers principles with keto, that's where you'll really get into trouble long term. Weight Watchers has been a sustainable business for decades for a reason - repeat customers.

So. Many. Repeat. Customers.

Sure, it might seem like smooth sailing at first, but I've seen many a ketoer get stuck without answers when following keto combined with Weight Watchers. Then this keto guru who led them down that path swears the ketoer must be doing something wrong.

These poor ketoers end up hungry and frustrated and fat. Again. Many of those who religiously follow Weight Watchers may notice a similar pattern of initial success, followed by a stall, followed by a return to poor diet habits and weight regain.

I'm here to help you get unstuck … or maybe never even fall into these keto traps in the first place. Never getting stuck in the first place sounds like a better idea.

Do I know everything there is to know about how every person should keto?

No. Making that claim is silly. We're all individuals, and that's why it's important to learn how to individualize a keto plan that's right for you.

You have a different preferred lifestyle and a different body chemistry than I have. Your previous diet and exercise history are also different from mine. Since all of these factors will go into how you should best keto, telling you to follow exactly the same plan I followed to lose more than 100 pounds won't work.

Well, it might work; but at the very least you'll have to make tweaks in order for the steps I took to work for you.

That doesn't even touch on the fact that my keto lifestyle changed so much along my 110 pound weight loss journey. It *had* to change in order for me to see continued success. Taking in the exact same macros and calories day after day for the rest of your keto life is another great way to find yourself in a big fat keto weight loss stall. That's also an easy way to get bored with this lifestyle.

My keto plan changed from the beginning to the middle, and again before the end.

Actually, the way I keto is ever evolving, even during my weight maintenance phase. That is one of the biggest reasons it's important for you to figure out how to individualize keto to your own unique body chemistry and digestive capabilities. You have to learn how to work with your body to help make keto work long term for you.

For those who say success lies only in macro counting, I see many of these people once they reach their goal weight. Mostly, I see their struggle.

Sure, they're all knowledge and smiles when it comes to telling you how they keto, but someday only focusing on macro counting and nothing else catches up with them. I watch with one eye covered as the weight slowly creeps back on, yet they still dish out the same tired "only focus on the macros" advice.

Since I'm a stay at home mom, I'm really only talking about a few people I've seen on Instagram who I've never actually met. Most of my mom friends I see in real life are too busy shuffling kids around to even think about whether or not the meals they eat on the fly are keto friendly. They typically only find time to shove whatever leftover toddler snacks they can find into their face before moving onto their next mom task.

No judgement - sometimes I'm about that life too.

While I know first hand my mom friends may have good intentions, organic Goldfish aren't exactly the health food Pepperidge Farm claims them to be. Yes, they make organic Goldfish. Don't ask me how I know.

All I'm trying to say is maybe *some people* can only count macros and still find long term success. Not everyone will put the weight back on because they didn't take time to improve some of the stuff I had to. If counting macros is the only thing you need to do for lasting success, keto on! I have no hate in my heart for those who can make keto as simple as adding up carbs.

For me, keto was never that simple. If you've tried keto or low carb plans in the past, and you also failed miserably, keto likely won't be that simple this time around for you either.

The good news is, the stories and information you're about to read in this book can help make keto *seem* easy for you; at least once you put in the grunt work.

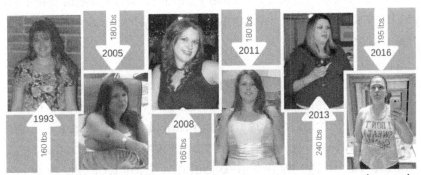

(Following every latest diet fad I came across - including many low carb plans that teach quick fixes instead of a real food approach, I constantly struggled with yo-yoing weight)

I finally took time to put in the work at the beginning of my low carb plan, before I ever moved onto keto, and I'm so happy I did!

Taking the steps I talk about in the next few chapters of this book not only helped me find success with the weight loss part of keto, but it also makes maintaining my 100 pound loss a breeze. Gone are the days where I struggle to stay in the same size, season after season.

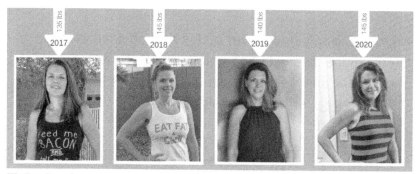

(Following the strategies I teach in this book, I no longer struggle to stay within a healthy weight range.)

I'm in a body I love, and it's been easy to maintain for the first time in my life. I've also experienced life changing health benefits. I've improved health issues I've had for years that I previously thought I was just stuck with. Heck, I even improved health conditions I didn't even know I had!

I guess this keto stuff is magic after all.

Yes, keto can be magical in the end if you follow a keto plan that's realistic and right for you. Eating real food that is high in fat, low in carbs and right for your chemistry can absolutely be magical. There are plenty of successful ketoers out there that can vouch for this!

Seriously, there are so many keto success stories! D'ya hear that, Jillian Michaels?

Maybe she just needs some feel good ketones in her life, because that chick is scary! Also, her workouts are unnecessarily hard. Also squared - I'd be curious to see some of her long term success stories.

'Cause me, I've got quite a few of my own stacking up!

Like Suzanne. She's down over 80 lbs and off several long term medications since starting keto in 2018. That loss took a little over a year and it's a loss she still maintains today. (She's in our membership, so we definitely K.I.T.)

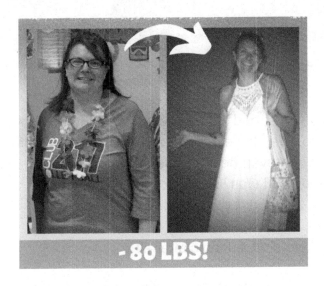

And we can't forget about one of my first coaching clients Alissa, who lost 58 lbs in 2017, reversed several health conditions, including fatty liver disease, and weaned off medications for type 2 diabetes, chronic heartburn and arthritis.

A lot of her progress was made in about four months of following keto the right way. Her husband shed 51 lbs in that same timeframe! I see them all the time on social media, and they're still doing great!

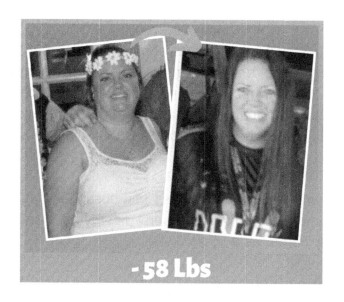

- 58 Lbs

I've witnessed plenty of other long term keto success stories of those who've had a completely life altering transformation in a short amount of time. I hear from so many who've easily maintained for the first time ever, including from several people who lost 100 pounds or more just from reading my books, so perhaps Jillian needs to shut her trap when it comes to how dangerous a real food diet like a keto plan is.

Oh right, that's something else I wanted to mention before we get into the meat of this book. (Meat ... see what I just did there?)

There are so many lessons I've learned throughout my keto journey that go against everything most of us have learned about diet and exercise. One of those things is everyone needs to work out unbelievably hard in order to get weight loss results.

I tried that route with pretty much every diet I've tried; didn't work.

Later in this book, I'll teach you how I *eat more* and *move less* for better weight loss results. As in, I eat way more - some days almost double what I ate on miserable starvation diets of the past. I also work out way less. In fact, for extended periods of my keto life, I didn't have time to work out at all. I still saw results.

There are plenty of other diet myths I'll be busting throughout this book; some keto and some general diet myths. I learned a ton during my career as a yo-yo dieter.

Unfortunately, most of that was all of the stuff not to do. Yet, like a sad hamster cruising along on her sad hamster wheel, I kept at the same things that never worked long term.

I've since learned a ton of brand new info over my six year low carb lifestyle.

Since I was able to successfully lose more than 100 pounds and actually maintain my loss this time around, you know, beyond that one year I gained *some* of the weight back in order to grow another human, I'd say what I learned this time around seems to be spot on. I'm so happy to have this opportunity to share the strategies that really work with you.

As a fellow dieter, I understand you want all of the weight loss deets, and you want them now! Even though I no longer believe in quick fix plans, I do believe you can start on the right path right this instant with my free guide, where I walk you through the five biggest secrets to my amazing weight loss success story.

That's not vain, is it? Calling my own story amazing?

I mean, losing more than 100 lbs and keeping it off for three years is pretty ah-mazing, am-I-right? It's a task more than 95% of people can't accomplish ... including some pretty big heavy hitters who have fancy chefs in their kitchens, personal trainers delivered to their doorsteps, and still get paid millions to promote popular diet programs.

Yep, the same popular diet programs we've all tried and failed a bazillion times ... and I'm even including the aforementioned heavy hitters in that 95% statistic, because even they've all regained everything they lost. So I don't believe I'm being vain by referring to my own story as amazing.

Vain or not, I really don't care if this song is about me. My vanity is in the name of helping you get results, so please allow me to Warren Beatty this book up so you can learn all of my secrets when it comes to my amazing weight loss success story.

Once you hit your goal, we can walk into the party together just like we were walking onto a yacht! It's a lot of fun, I swear.

(Hitting your goal weight is fun, not walking onto a yacht. Indie authors on Amazon just don't got it like that.)

So about those secrets I mentioned before I dished the dirt on who Carly Simon was actually singing about in her early 70's smash hit ...

Definitely keep reading this book since it contains a lot of helpful info you can use for *your* keto success story; but you can also get a sneak peek of the tactics I talk about with my free guide.

In the guide, I share the five biggest secrets to my success ... secrets I still use today to maintain my loss. Oh, and if you're still in a hurry, the guide talks about the five strategies I used to lose five pants sizes in only five months.

The guide is a solid high five to your success! (Wow, I promise not to cheese out like that again.)

You can get that free guide here.

Now, before we get to how my life began in this low carb world, let's take the next chapter to talk about one of the biggest keto myths of all: let's chit chat about the fat.

In particular, what happened to all of the fat on keto? There are many a keto expert out there telling everyone to cut fat from their high fat diets, and it really bugs me. I get even more fired up when their audience is made up of women who spent a lifetime in the diet world, like me. For these women, no advice could be worse.

So really, where's the fat?

Chapter 1: Where's the Fat?

I looked up keto in the dictionary, because after almost seven years of following this lifestyle with a lot of success, even I'm confused. I thought maybe looking it up on good old *Webster's* might help clear up some of my confusion.

Of course, when people talk about the dictionary these days, most of us mean Google, right? Is there anyone out there who actually still uses a paperback dictionary? Because I'm a writer with a moldy brain, and I don't even have one of those. More on that moldy brain stuff to come. It's a doozy!

Back to the true meaning of keto. Merriam Webster tells us keto means, "of or relating to a ketone." Using a word to define that word … yep, Merriam is just as confused as the rest of us! We really shouldn't trust anyone named Merriam anyway. She sounds so high-flutant and stuffy.

Apologies to my former roommate whose name was also Merriam. Even though you're a sweet girl, your name is high-flutant and stuffy.

Wikipedia does a little better with it's keto definition. Wikipedia defines keto as, "a high fat, adequate-protein, low carbohydrate diet…" and goes on to talk about the ketogenic diet in relation to epileptic children.

Right, because that's how ketogenic diets began back in the 1920's. These diets weren't used for weight loss at all. Food was used as medicine to help control epilepsy in children. Ah, the good old days when doctors were professionals who sought out cures for their patients with actual protocols that work instead of masking current symptoms with drugs that cause new symptoms. Food is medicine. I know I've heard that somewhere.

Yes, I'm a tad jaded when it comes to the medical industry. Twenty years of doctor's visits with only temporary relief for my symptoms, with a whole new host of symptoms arising, can do that to a girl.

Of course, sometimes the natural medical community isn't all that much better, as I learned a few years ago. While attempting to fix up some lingering health issues, I spent several thousand dollars to be told to eat more fish. When I sought out additional help, I was advised to drink more bone broth.

A girl can't live on bone broth and fish alone, little lone expect to heal on a diet made up of mostly bone broth and fish.

Well, maybe that works. I refuse to eat anything from the sea, so even with my best efforts put forth, I never quite figured out if the solution I paid more than $7,000 for actually works. A tiny piece of the puzzle the doctor helped me unearth led to my eventual path of healing, so I'll still call that medical debacle a win.

OK, so Merriam, who's supposed to be the gold standard when it comes to definitions, confuses us more, while Wikipedia, who's run by the masses, does a much better job.

Sounds about right to me! Let's say Wikipedia is correct, and we call keto a high fat diet. Assuming this is the correct definition, where's the fat?

I keep seeing keto advocate after keto advocate telling us to quit eating so much fat on a high fat diet. I do believe these keto advocates seem to be getting their education from stuffy Merriam, because they're confusing everyone who's just starting out on keto by telling them to limit fat on their high fat diets.

Now I'm not saying everyone should be melting coconut oil and chugging it throughout the day, because yuck; but telling people to eat low fat on a high fat diet … um, does anyone else see a problem with this?

You might be confused since many of these 'experts' don't necessarily use the words "eat low fat." They still want you to eat high fat foods like avocados and olive oil, but only if you carefully monitor calories at the same time.

I know back in my yo-yoing days, I counted every single calorie that entered my mouth. During the weeks or months I went rogue and tried low carb again, it was basically so I could get a break from counting calories. It was so I could feel good again by providing my body food.

I did feel fabulous … for at least a few weeks because I saw results, and I was able to eat food. I never connected the feeling fabulous part with eating enough food, or even with eating real food, because that's a big part of it as well.

If you know anything about me, you know I've been trying low carb diets since the late 90's. This was when the taboo Atkins Diet was making a triumphant return. I went on and off of the Atkins Diet many times between 1998 - 2014. I never stuck with it long term for several reasons.

The biggest reason was after spending so much time dieting via low calorie methods, my body didn't digest fat or protein very well. This also happened because I grew up in the generation that ate plenty of the government recommended 'healthy' whole grain carbs. Snackwell low-fat cookies and baked potato chips replaced my higher fat favorites because they were lower in fat and calories.

I even tried Olestra chips for a hot minute … which resulted in a hot trip to the toilet every time. Hot, as in burning diarrhea. How did that stuff ever get FDA approval?

I also didn't love to cook. I lived in Chicago where there's a hot dog stand every ten feet. The smell of french fries were often too overwhelming to resist for very long. When you mix the aroma of hot dog joints with the exhaustion I felt while starving my body of nutrients, let's just say that wasn't a winning combo for lasting success.

Sure, I was eating more food than I typically allowed myself on low calorie diets, which was great … but I was still pretty exhausted since once I burned through my glycogen stores, which came from the carbs I ate while eating low calorie, (or still snuck in while 'low carb'). I didn't have any fuel for my body since it no longer digested fat or protein in a super effective manner.

When you feel like you've been run over by a mack truck day after day on your low carb diet because you're not providing your body with fuel it can actually use, you tend to not stick to your low carb diet very long. This was my life. And then, I was back to counting calories, even while following a low carb plan.

The Truth About Calories In vs. Calories Out

Even though this method failed me time and again, I figured I'd give it another try since that's what the mainstream tells us to do. Move more, eat less and weight loss success shall be yours.

They leave out the part where you'll need to keep moving even more and eating even less until you're basically falling apart from malnutrition when you follow this method ... you know, if you'd like to prevent weight regain.

This was also my life - the falling apart part.

The list of health issues I experienced over my twenty year yo-yo diet history can fill a book. Oh wait, that's part of what you'll read about in this book. But I'll also tell you how I improved all of these health issues, so don't feel like I'm only using my misery to keep you company.

I followed the mainstream advice about moving more and eating less. In fact, I was an A+ student. Once the experts brought calorie counting to keto, I bought a first class ticket aboard that train too because keto seemed to be magical and *everybody knows you must eat low calorie in order to lose weight*. (I'm saying that in my best Phaedra Parks accent. Shout out old school RHOA fans).

I thought I found a winning combo that was foolproof. Turns out, I was the fool for continuing to fall for the biggest myth we all still believe about weight loss: *calories in versus calories out*.

Yes CICO is a myth. Yes, you probably believe this myth. Don't feel bad since you are far from alone in your beliefs.

We all stopped believing in Santa Claus long ago, right? Can calorie counting please hitch a sleigh ride to the North Pole on Rudolph's back and stay there? Well, perhaps not Rudolph. He's had a hard enough time as it is.

What about Donner or Blitzen? What are they doing to earn their keep these days?

Now everyone can clearly see the jolly fat man in red isn't in any danger of falling into the calorie counting trap with all of his high sugar milk and cookies, so let's just fly this method off with him and his reindeer, and leave it to die a cold and icy death.

If you're still a hardcore believer in this method, you have two choices. One choice is you can stick your fingers in your ears while screaming, "La, la, la." While that may be your preference, it won't work.

This is mostly due to the fact that you're reading a book. I'm a mere indie health author, and likely not popular enough to have this recorded as an audiobook. Even if someday my writing does become that popular, I know it might feel more like we're having a conversation, but I still can't hear you.

If you really don't want to learn what I have to say, the least you'll have to do is cover your eyes since I won't hear your screams. In fact, you're probably still in the sample portion of this e-book. You could also just not click the "Buy Now" option, because that would work too.

I'm 100% ok with telling you not to buy my book. There's enough keto crazies in the world telling me that I have no clue how this weight loss stuff works, even though I struggled through their methods for two decades with zero lasting success.

Keto crazies from all over the world tell me I don't know what I'm talking about, even though I went on to lose more than 100 pounds, easily zipped right past my goal, and have somehow managed to keep more than 100 pounds off for over three years.

Nope, I haven't a clue. (insert eye roll)

In fact, I happen to be a magical fairy who struggled with weight loss for most of her life, and then one day the Weight Loss Gods decided to do me a solid, and humbly allowed all of my nonsensical methods to work … but just for me, and just this one time.

They felt so much pity for my situation that they even allowed me to maintain my huge loss. I suppose the Weight Loss Gods felt sorry for me after noticing the hard work I put in for so many years with the tried and true weight loss methods that are *guaranteed* to work for every other person on the planet, like eating less calories than you burn.

That's how *all* of us Americans maintain spectacular health and completely normal weights, right?

Only, I never found lasting success with this method, even while simultaneously eating keto macros. The Weight Loss Gods sprinkled their magical weight loss dust on me and poof! I lost 90 pounds after my first pregnancy, and another 65 pounds after my second with methods that clearly work for no one. Except me. Just this one time.

Surely since the methods I talk about are hogwash that work for no one, someday soon I'll wake up to 100 pounds of regained weight. Right? Any day now?

Yep, still waiting.

That was a really long made up story all to say that people on the keto message boards are mean, and perhaps after researching all of this health and weight loss stuff for several years, maybe I know a thing or two about a thing or two after all. Maybe I am smart enough to realize that we're all different, and no one plan will work for every person out there. Maybe.

If you're done shoving your fingers in your ears and screaming at someone that can't hear you, there's another option. Perhaps you can have an open mind when it comes to the insanity that is calorie counting, while also constantly trying to burn more calories off than you take in from day to day.

Perhaps you can finally start to see keto as a diet where you burn fat based on hormones, rather than a plan where you not only need to monitor every single calorie you shove into your mouth, but now you have to add in complicated math equations and percentages to figure out precise ratios of the calorie macros you take in.

Maybe you can even see keto as a plan where, at times, you actually require extra fat coming in so your body that is overstressed from too many years of calorie deprivation finally realizes it's safe enough to let go of some of your stored body fat.

Before keto hit the streets, the name of the weight loss game was mainly calories in versus calories out. Now that we've added keto to the mix, so many out there not only want you to focus on calories, but they also want you to calculate the exact percentage of carbs, protein and fat you fit into your calorie range as well.

And even though this is a keto diet, which we've already defined as a high fat diet; since you have fat on your body to burn, you don't want to waste that opportunity by taking in any extra nutritional fat.

Not. Even. An. Ounce.

While that logic can maybe be correct in specific circumstances, there's a time and a place for it, and at the start of your keto diet is not the time, nor the place.

If you find success with keto following this logic at the start, you're actually not following a keto diet at all. You're back to a calories in versus calories out model, and you don't even know it because you're allowing yourself to dine on extra delicious fat at the expense of your beloved carbs.

You've been told to raise your fat, but only a little, and then lower your carbs drastically to compensate. The experts who tout this logic tell you once you get these two aspects correct, you're golden.

You've been bamboozled into thinking you're automatically in ketosis whenever you cut carbs below 20 and you keep calories low. Now the weight is sure to fall off each and every week - guaranteed.

At least until it doesn't.

While you may show ketones at this stage of the diet game, especially on those pretty purple pee sticks, please know these are starvation ketones, and starvation ketones won't lead to the results you want long term.

While you may show pounds lost on the scale at this stage of the diet game, keep in mind a lot of the weight you're losing from effectively starving yourself is coming from a loss of water due to dropping your carbohydrate intake, plus some bone and muscle loss thrown in for good measure.

Oh, that's right. A body that feels like it's being starved won't focus on making stronger bones or more muscle to help you age in a healthy manner.

A body that feels like it's being starved will use the muscle you already have on your body as energy. Since your body is being starved of enough nutrients coming in just to function, it really has no choice. Your body either needs to eat away at your muscle, or you will die ... or perhaps something less dramatic.

So maybe you followed this low calorie keto method, and maybe you lost 10 pounds on the scale. Hooray for dehydration and a body that's wasting away to nothing at a slow pace! Keto on!

According to a lot of keto experts out there, or at least many ketoers on the message boards who successfully lost 10 or 15 pounds on their keto plans (so of course they suddenly know everything there is to know about how a ketogenic diet works for every single person on the planet), all you need to get into ketosis is to drop your carbs below 20 per day. Eat less than 20 carbs each day and watch the fat melt away!

Hey, that even sounds a little catchy.

The catchy advice is as long as you drop carbs, the weight will fall right off. These keto overachievers approached their keto plans this way and lost weight, which means every person on the planet should get to their goal weight by eating less than 20 carbs each day.

Easy peasy; end of story.

If you follow this method, and you don't lose weight via this one easy dietary change, you're clearly exceeding your 20 carbs per day goal. If you tell these message board experts you're not exceeding your 20 carb goal, you are clearly a big fat carb consuming liar.

Following this same social media logic, if someone who has a weekly keto podcast and has written four books on the subject, so perhaps she may call herself a bit of a keto expert by this point, tries to steer these unfortunate ketoers down the same path she used to lose more than 100 pounds, but maybe there was a little more to her story than someone on social media who goes by the name of TracyandBrian says the story should be, TracyandBrian will hunt this helpful ketoer down.

TracyandBrian will stalk her and berate her until they wear her down enough to admit she's a big fat liar! Their end goal is to make her concede that while she did in fact lose more than 100 pounds following a low carb lifestyle, all she had to do was lower her carbs to below 20 because THERE IS NO OTHER WAY.

Someone on social media named TracyandBrian succeeded by only lowering carbs below 20 grams, and if he or she, because I still haven't quite figured out if I'm being berated by the Tracy portion of this account, or the Brian portion, but if he or she finds out anyone ever succeeded any other way than by only lowering carbs to under 20 each day - YOU ARE WRONG because THERE IS NO OTHER WAY.

TracyandBrian is always ready to pounce with his or her slew of science backed articles. TracyandBrian is prepared to shove these articles down your throat at a moment's notice to prove he or she is right.

Seriously - does anyone know this TracyandBrian person? Is it a he or a she?

My guess is it's a she because I can't think of too many men with their man goodies still attached that would agree to troll Facebook as hardcore as TracyandBrian does with a joint marital account.

I apologize if you too have a joint marital Facebook account. I just assumed we were all supposed to trust the person we married a little bit more than forcing a joint Facebook account. At the very least, spy on your partner's solo account in secrecy like a decent human being. Don't put on display to the entire world how little you trust your spouse by forcing a joint marital account.

So did this TracyandBrian method work for you? And if so, why are you here reading yet another diet book written by a girl who admittedly comes off a bit snarky at times?

Are you hate reading this book? Definitely let me know if I'm popular enough to have hate readers, because that would be pretty cool.

Or maybe you enjoy getting yelled at while you're just trying to lose weight for the love of the Weight Loss Gods.

Ok, I'll never yell at you. None of this is really all that serious to me. And while I have no controlled scientific studies to shove down your throat, please understand that my snark comes from love, and my research comes from too many years of trying far too many methods that failed me.

All of these failed methods did teach me that while perhaps they worked for someone at some point, that someone was not me.

Also, regarding the snark - I might at times find myself humorous, and I occasionally laugh out loud at my own dry sense of humor. I know that's not how dry humor works, but I eat a lot of fat, which results in a lot of feel good ketones.

Sometimes I just feel giddy, even when it comes to dry jokes that no one else LOL's at.

If you can relate, we'll be fast friends.

Even if you're not a fan of humor in the diet books you devour, you may still want to keep reading because I have an entire book coming at you filled with keto troubleshooting methods that may finally help you figure out how to succeed on keto without really trying.

Chapter 2: Fix your S.A.D.ness with a K.I.S.S.

Transitioning from the Standard American Diet to low carb by Keeping it Super Simple

Perhaps you already know a little bit about my S.A.D. yo-yo diet history. If you haven't read any of my other books, and you haven't been fortunate enough to hear me share far too many stories I probably shouldn't feel comfortable sharing on podcasts, then please note, I'm a veteran of the dieting world for more than two decades. I've attempted, failed, and then reattempted a good chunk of mainstream diets in existence.

For far too long I sought out diet after diet, desperately searching for *the* magic diet that would not only help me take weight off, but also keep it off.

If you find yourself in a similar position where you still rely on mainstream tactics, pay attention to this tough love right here.

Stop! Just please staaahhppp!

The fitness industry is an 88 billion dollar industry for a reason. Quit buying what the mainstream is selling. You're a mere pauper contributing to their massive bottom line.

For those who think I'm exaggerating, or maybe you think you've got me beat when it comes to who's tried the most diets, let's take a walk down memory lane, and revisit all of my diets from Christmas past.

Indulge me these next few minutes to reminisce about some of the mainstream plans I've failed miserably over the past few decades.

My S.A.D. Existence

SlimFast

My first gateway into the dieting world was with SlimFast. If I can recall correctly, I snuck my first can of chocolate SlimFast while babysitting four boys under age eight when I was only twelve.

I had zero business babysitting four rambunctious boys, as I was still a kid myself. I also had zero business drinking weight loss shakes as a snack, followed by chips and frozen pizza for dinner.

The chocolate shake I drank in secret tasted pretty good. My naive preteen self was under the impression that just drinking a can of this stuff every now and then would help with weight loss. Little did I know, SlimFast had an entire *starve yourself by drinking these shakes as meals so you very un-heathily lose weight plan* to go along with it.

Seriously, one shake of liquid sugars for breakfast, one shake of liquid sugars for lunch, followed by a small dinner consisting of low fat meat mixed with rabbit clippings isn't sustainable for anyone long term.

By rabbit clippings, I mean iceberg salad mixed with shredded carrots, plus a tasteless low calorie, low fat dressing on the side. That's what I think you're supposed to eat ... at least according to Whoopi, the only celebrity SlimFast spokesperson I can remember.

You definitely aren't supposed to eat a Big Mac meal with a Diet Coke as your sensible dinner. I can tell you first hand, that SlimFast plan does not work.

As an adult, I moved onto low carb SlimFast, which didn't taste nearly as delicious as its high sugar counterpart.

When I followed low carb back in the day, there weren't as many quick and easy low carb convenience foods. Since I had zero clue how to cook, I was all about the quick and easy convenience foods.

Now they even market a Keto SlimFast, which I will not be trying. I actually joked about Keto SlimFast before there was ever such a product ... and then a few months later SlimFast contacted me on Instagram to ask if I had interest in becoming a Keto SlimFast ambassador. I couldn't believe this product I spoke of in jest became a real product just a few months later.

If you've taken our Virtual Coaching Course, you probably recall I talked about using *The Secret*, as in the book, to envision your goals. I just want the universe to be clear when I joked about Keto SlimFast, that was not me envisioning a Keto SlimFast drink. While it's good to know secreting really works, I'd prefer to use these magical powers for good instead of evil.

LA Weight Loss

Moving right along to more crazy diets I've tried over the years ...

One time, and only one time, I tried LA Weight Loss. I feel the need to qualify that with 'only one time' because with most of these other plans, I tried them, failed miserably, and for some reason they'd actually work for me this time around if I tried them again.

In case you haven't heard of LA Weight Loss, this is a plan where you make appointments at their centers a few times each week for consultations. You weigh in each time you make an appearance. They also make you buy their weight loss bars that taste eerily similar to a candy bar. They must have been magical candy bars due to their astronomical price tag per bar.

It's been awhile since I've been, but I remember some type of insanely low calorie plan as part of the deal. I didn't last too long with LA Weight Loss, even after spending a small fortune to start the plan, because who really has time to hit up a center to weigh in three times each week?

I think they sold the pit-stops as accountability, but looking back I honestly believe visiting three times each week was a tactic to upsell more magical weight loss candy bars.

Weight Watchers

Then there's Weight Watchers, a low calorie plan I've tried too many times to count. I will admit here that I've only tried Weight Watchers Online, so I can't vouch for the in person experience.

I never attended in person meetings ever since being scared off by how a meeting was portrayed on *Sex and the City*.

If you saw the episode where Miranda's weight gets screwed up, and then called out in front of everyone at the meeting, I'm sure you're with me here.

Sure, these days I blast my weight on message boards all over social media alongside a scantily clothed photo; but back in my yo-yo days when my weight wasn't stable, and it was a number I was deeply ashamed of, that number was more closely guarded than Monica's infamous blue dress with the mysterious white stain.

(R.I.P. Linda Tripp. While your intentions were sketchy, you deserved every last piece of notoriety you gained for guarding that semen stained dress so closely ... because really, who else would risk touching Bill Clinton's infamous white and gooey for a little good ole fashioned blackmail?)

Not even the frightening political machine that is the Clintons could have pried that secret out of my clammy, puffy hands.

While I never attended a meeting, the amount of times I started and stopped Weight Watchers Online was enough to single handedly inspire Oprah to invest in the company.

It's also important to note the amount of pounds I've lost and regained with Weight Watchers Online is enough to fill Oprah's infamous red wagon of fat at least ten times over.

Jenny Craig

I also gave Jenny Craig a few whirls in my 20's and 30's. During my very first J-Craig attempt, even way back before Kirstie Alley was losing and regaining weight with the plan as a paid spokesperson, I lived with a few roommates in Chicago where three of us shared a small freezer. I'm almost positive my roomies were none too excited the first time I came home with dozens of tiny frozen meals Jenny Craig requires you to buy from their centers each week.

Looking back, I can see where our roommate love story began to unfold. (We didn't exactly end our living situation on good terms) It all makes sense now since I took up the entire freezer with frozen mini-meals that were supposed to have the weight falling off.

At the detriment of my friendships, I did lose weight with the meals. I struggled when it came time to add the real food portion of the plan, like vegetables alongside the frozen meals, because my palette was so accustomed to consuming the highly processed foods they sold. Once it came time to eat anything that wasn't chemically produced in a lab, I really wanted no part of the real food they promoted buying alongside their packaged meals. Especially with low fat, tasteless ranch dressing … because yuck!

I struggled with Jenny Craig because, as is the case with most of these mainstream plans, I was *f'ing hungry!*

I'd eventually lose interest in going to the centers to weigh in and buy more food and before I knew it, I spiraled off my mainstream plan face first into a fried food sampler from Bennigans.

Right about now I'm sure you're thinking, "You mean the same appetizer that's meant for the entire table to share? That Bennigan's sampler?"

Yep, there were many days I considered the entire platter lunch. And once I drowned all of my diet sorrows in every last spring roll, it was onward and upward to the next flashy fad.

More than a few times I even tried my own homemade version of Jenny Craig where I figured out the amount of calories the center had me consume, and then I'd buy the same types of meals, like Lean Cuisines, to make up my own knock off version.

I was still ravenous most of the time, so even my poor man's version of Jenny Craig never lasted long before I ditched my calorie counting ways for a cheap and addictive fast food lunch.

I always went into restaurants during my lunch break with the best intentions of getting something low calorie and low fat, but once the amazing smell of fried foods infiltrated my brain, I swear, I blacked out.

Even with weight loss desperation always at the forefront of my mind, I somehow mysteriously awoke face first in the lettuce drippings leftover from my double cheeseburger. Every. Single. Time.

It was a vicious cycle.

Pricey Diet Coach

When I was fed up with attempting to 'go it alone' in my mid 20's, I enlisted the help of a diet coach I saw on the news. I fought city traffic to meet her at her downtown condo where she took my measurements, and we covered what I should eat. She was pricey, but since she offered to come grocery shopping with me, I thought she was well worth the price. What other diet programs offered field trips as part of the package?

During our grocery store soiree, my new skinny Minnie coach pointed out meals like Lean Cuisines, which of course I was already familiar with, but she let me know these teensy meals weren't actually meant for one as their labels imply.

My pricey skinny Minnie friend let me in on her secret to success. On her plan, she split Lean Cuisine meals with her husband, and then added a small side salad for each of them.

Is this why I never found Jenny Craig success? Did my coaches lead me astray by making me believe these meals were meant for one, when these microwaveable, frozen delights were really meant for two all along?

Looking back, I'm not exactly sure why I paid this woman big bucks to tell me to eat half of a Lean Cuisine. While I did have the ability to call her anytime I was in danger of going off my plan, with only half a Lean Cuisine as nourishment, I was pretty much always in danger of going off my plan.

Low Carb and Macro Counting

I don't want these mainstream diets to be the only plans that get a bad rap, because trust- you-me, I also tried some version of a low carb diet many, many times since my late teens.

I followed Atkins dating back all the way to the late 90's. Back in the day, I had a boyfriend who was obsessed with nutrition, and he was on a quest for the perfect body. He found Atkins, and being ever the devoted and love-smitten girlfriend, I was completely on board to join him.

Well, at least for a few meals. In the back of my mind, I was deathly afraid of having a heart attack in my teens since that's what the mainstream warned would happen with a 'fad diet' like Atkins.

I tried some version of a low carb diet again in my younger 20's with a few friends at work. I can still remember being absolutely dumbfounded by losing 9 lbs in less than three weeks.

Losing 9 lbs in only 3 weeks!?!? Have you ever heard of such a miracle?

Of course these days my Keto Challengers have been known to lose up to 25 lbs in only three weeks, but I will admit, that's just me being a braggy coach.

And for the sake of keeping it real, only one challenger has made it to that 25 lb mark … but many others lose 10, 15, even up to 20 lbs in only 21 days! I think with results like that, I have the right to be at least a little braggy.

But back to my early low carb days.

The friends I tried my latest low carb attempt with worked with me in the mortgage industry. This was the mid-2000's, not too much earlier than the entire industry collapsed because of all of the loan shenanigans going down.

That alone should clue you into how stressed we all were. The fact that we worked at a company owned by a brother sister duo who must have grown up in an extremely dysfunctional household did not help our situation. We spent many lunch breaks stress eating burgers without the buns.

As is common when it comes to newbies following low carb plans they don't understand, the buns, plus a loaded side of fries, found their place back onto all of our plates. The weight we lost also quickly returned, plus more.

I also followed the *Protein Power* book, *The South Beach Diet,* which is more of a Mediterranean plan where you also cut back on carbs, and the *Zone Diet*, where you have to calculate your meals to macro percentages of 40/30/30.

I did tons of macro calculating and calorie counting for years. I now have the ability to look at pretty much any serving of food, and I can tell you the exact calories in it. I guess you can call me a calorie savant.

Diet Pills

Despite Jessie Spano's terrifying warnings in *Saved by the Bell*, I also tested out diet pills.

One of my favorite hobbies back in the day was strolling the aisle of Walgreens in search of some kind of pill that would curb my appetite so I could finally shed pounds without constant hunger.

I ordered fancy, and most likely dangerous, weight loss supplements from the internet. I even found a doctor that prescribed Phentermine for just about anyone who wanted it, so I tried that for a while.

The prescription for Phentermine actually did control my appetite for a few months, so I did find some initial success. None of the over the counter stuff really did much beyond making me feel jittery.

With the prescribed stuff, I felt more in control and lost weight. Of course I had to spend hundreds of dollars to take a slew of medical tests to get the stuff, but I thought all of the effort was worth the success I had with these prescription pills. Plus, if a doctor agreed I needed them, surely they were safe and necessary, right?

Eventually it was shown this medication, or some version of it, was killing people. The FDA started cracking down and it became nearly impossible to get. Even though the medication was resulting in death, it was working for me and I wanted my fix.

Looking back, it's really sad to think that I risked my health and basically my life just to find something that reduced my appetite.

In all honesty, I'm not sure anyone really knows I took that drug beyond a few friends I worked with at the time. They only knew since I ran into them at the doctor's office since they were taking it too. We all kept it hush, hush as our little secret.

I hid it from everyone else because I didn't want anyone to judge me for taking a weight loss drug. Deep down, I knew it was probably doing bad things to my body; I must have known since I kept it a secret.

CICO (Calories In vs. Calories Out)

The diet plan I followed the most over my twenty year struggle was cutting calories very low while over exercising with cardio at least 6-7 days per week.

I typically spent about an hour on cardio machines most days. Sometimes I wasted upwards of 90 minutes or more.

There's a term for this type of lifestyle called Orthorexia. This disease is when someone displays an obsession with eating foods that one considers healthy. To me, healthy was anything that could help me keep calories low. I over exercised to stay in a caloric deficit, or so I thought.

I'm confident there were many other diets I followed over my 20 year yo-yo history, but then you'd be here all day reading about all of the diets that failed me.

At some point, I'd like to get to how you can go from this world where you're struggling and hopping from diet to diet, to a place where this all just becomes natural and easy.

I want to help get you to a place where you no longer have to diet because you're just a happy ketoer living your best keto lifestyle.

Is Keto A Fad?

Fad diets are defined as: a diet that is popular for a time, similar to fads in fashion.
I'd classify many of the diets I tried over the years as fads.

Fad diets usually promise rapid weight loss or other health advantages, such as a longer life. They are often promoted as requiring little effort and producing a 'quick fix.'

There are many who refer to keto and low carb as fads, which is interesting since we've eaten real food as a species since pretty much the dawn of man. Back in the day, like back in the caveman days, our ancestors ran on ketones much of the time.

I suppose you could classify keto as a fad if you go into it with the intention of a quick fix plan where you will only drop carbs for a limited time, and then you plan to go back to eating the same junk that got you into your current situation.

I can tell you right now, most people who go into keto with that attitude won't last long.

Keto isn't an easy diet if you start with that attitude. While low carb is a little easier than keto, it's also not an easy diet if you look at it as something you will only follow as a quick fix solution until you hit your goal.

Low carb definitely isn't a fad diet for me considering I've been following low carb as a lifestyle since early 2014, and I moved onto keto in early 2015.

In all honesty, I didn't know low carb would become my lifestyle when I started dropping carbs in 2014. I was like many dieters out there. I wanted to lose weight fast, and I was willing to do whatever it took, even if that meant ditching all of the overly processed 'food-like' products that made up the bulk of my diet.

While I was desperate to lose weight, I had a bit of a dilemma since I also loved carbs. Even calling out my love affair with French fries and potato chips doesn't paint my relationship with carbs in the correct light.

I was a full blown carb addict. I couldn't fathom a life worth living if I couldn't live it with my daily bread.

I fully admit, I went into low carb with intentions for this approach to stick around long enough to drop the excess pounds. But this time around, I can say it finally stuck since here we are six years later, and I still successfully live a low carb lifestyle.

Guess what else happened! I finally got out of that viscous yo-yo diet cycle, while also escaping the awful diet mentality I was stuck in for decades.

Escaping Diet CULT-ure

Maybe I've been watching too much _Scientology and The Aftermath_ these days, but I feel like diet mentality is a cult. There are so many rules to follow, and you end up giving all of your money to the Diet Gods in order to reach an ultimate fate very few reach.

I'd like to say you're also seeking better health, but the sad truth is most of these diets that keep you stuck in diet mentality are doing everything *but* making you healthier. Twenty plus years of hopping from diet to diet left my health in absolute shambles.

I can confidently tell you this after that list of diets I just went through destroyed my health over the twenty plus years I followed them.

My journey into constant yo-young weight all began back in the early 90's when I cut fat out of my diet, since that was our diet savior then. I guess none of the experts of the 90's understood that our brains thrive on healthy fats, and we need healthy fats to feel good and for overall health.

I cut fat down to under 20 grams per day per their advice. That's when many of my health problems began.

Strange coincidence, eh?

(I threw that *eh* in for my Canadian readers. While I'm a mere indie author, I'm an indie author with worldwide reach thanks to the genius of Amazon.)

Let's chat about the easy steps I took to finally escape diet culture for good, and how I easily transitioned from the Standard American Diet of junk food for most meals, to a lifestyle that was lower in junk carbs.

This is the exact plan I followed to jumpstart weight loss and improve my health.

A lot of plans out there advise you to go all in. Even a lot of keto experts instruct you to jump straight into the deep end right away. They advise you to lower carbs below 20 right from the start, and then dive head first into healthy fats in order to reach the keto promised-land.

While I admire a lot of these experts, and I've learned a ton from them, that's not an approach I recommend.

Looking back at that girl who struggled with her health for so long, if I tried this method of jumping right in and going full on keto from the start - I would have failed miserably.

I'm sure I would have felt just fine the first few days, but by the time the weekend hit, my desperate carb cravings would have led to failure. And when you eat as much fat as is recommended on keto, and then you cheat on the weekend with carbs, you won't lose weight. In fact, this is *the best method* for weight gain.

If you continue to start each and every week with the best intentions, but continue falling off at some point during the week, or even if you hold out until the weekend, you're in another vicious cycle.

At this point, most people blame themselves.

You think you're doing something wrong. You feel dieter's guilt, which leads to you berating and punishing yourself. So you restrict calories more. You exercise even harder. You may even attempt to lower carbs even lower than 20 per day. But no matter how hard you try to keto, you always seem to end up in the same place.

If you find yourself in this cycle, I know exactly how you think and the actions you'll take because for so long I was you.

I tried the all or nothing diet approaches for years. I never found lasting success with these restrictive approaches.

There are a few factors that helped me finally come around from this cycle of self abuse. If you still struggle with following a low carb or keto diet, I want you to forget everything you've been taught and everything you've tried up until this point. Start from scratch with this very simple approach.

If you're struggling, stop attempting to drop carbs to under 20 right from the start. If you continue to follow this same all or nothing pattern week after week, or even if you can make it a little longer, but eventually fall off and end up binging on carbs, please quit blaming yourself. I want you to understand it's not your fault. This struggle comes down to physiology.

Your physiology is something stronger than you can control, and you likely won't find success with low carb or keto until you take time to work with your physiology, instead of forcing tactics your body isn't ready for.

Most people coming to keto right from the standard American diet do not have physiology that is primed for a ketogenic lifestyle. Basically, you've spent your entire life running off of glucose as fuel. If you suddenly take all of your glucose away by taking all of your carbs away, your body will freak out because it doesn't know how to run primarily off of fat.

If you spent years dieting with methods like strict calorie reduction, or you've attempted any of the fad diets I mentioned earlier, I have bad news.

At this point you need to understand your body most likely isn't digesting fat very well.

If you stopped eating healthy fats because your low calorie diet guru told you that's how to achieve weight loss, and you did this for a considerable amount of time; once you reintroduce healthy fats back into your plan, your body will still search for carbs to burn as fuel.

Quick burning carbs are all it understands how to burn effectively. Many of the healthy fats you're attempting to eat on your low carb plan will be stored as toxins - which means you get even fatter.

So now you've taken away all of your carbs, and you're forcing your body to run mostly on a fuel source it doesn't remember how to process. How do you think you'll feel at this point?

If you've tried and failed with keto in the past, you probably know you'll feel miserable. This is the reason your body is crying out for carbs by the weekend - it's physiology.

Your body knows how to run on glucose in an effective manner. Now that you took all of the glucose away, you screwed your body over. Your body will cuss you out until you give it what it can burn.

Eventually, your physiology will win and you'll binge on every last carb you can shove into your face. Then you'll become reacquainted with that same old song and dance where you blame yourself for cheating on a diet you never really stood a chance against in the first place.

There's an easier way to prime your body for low carb livin'

You're gearing up to read about the strategies I used throughout this book, so you're off to a great start! (I understand that was a long winded intro ... but I have a husband and two kids who never stop talking. I too need an outlet to get all of my words in each day.)

If you want to learn how I got off to a really easy start with my low carb lifestyle, and you need a little more help than a book can provide, I did put a Keto Kickstart Course together - and it's free!

Most experts have you jump all in, and then leave you to fly solo. Our goal is to be there to help you weave past all of the tree branches you might fly face first into along the way. The general gist of getting started with a low carb plan is for those who are new, or those who've had trouble sticking with low carb plans in the past, you can start by eating up to 25 carbs at each meal. This provides you much more flexibility than only 20 carbs per day, like most keto plans recommend.

You can even have a snack or two with carbs while allowing your body time to adjust to eating less carbs and more fat. Keep those snacks low in carbs too; maybe 15 or less carbs per snack.

Instead of rushing straight into an all real food plan that you may not love right now, start making swaps overtime. Don't go grocery shopping and fill your cart to the brim with strange produce you intend to eat, but you'll just end up throwing away because *A. you don't know how to cook it* and *B. you just don't want to eat it.*

I do recommend buying at least some new real foods you may not currently eat to allow your body a chance to learn how to live on real food over time, but don't feel like you need to do everything all at once. Take appropriate steps to make this your lifestyle, not another diet you're forcing yourself to follow.

It might be a good idea to still buy some of your favorite foods that are lower in carbs, but understand your goal is to wean yourself off over time. Most experts won't recommend this, but I'm also guessing these experts don't remember how hard it can be starting out on a real food plan when you're coming from a place where most of the food you eat is processed.

Either they don't remember, or they never lived that life in the first place. I've definitely been there - done that, and I remember how much I depended on processed foods for day-to-day life.

When I tried the all or nothing approaches starting out, I failed miserably; each and every time. I understand the need to start swapping foods out overtime in order to make this lifestyle work for many people, including myself.

Wean If You Need Time to Wean

When I first began my low carb lifestyle, if I had a craving for fries - I ate them; but I was sure to limit them to only a few, and then filled up on the lower carb foods I needed to eat in order to find success. I continued to eat my processed junk favorites less and less, until I realized I felt much better by avoiding them all together. With taking the steps to improve the way my body digested food, I finally arrived at a place where my body was able to use some of the other food sources I was giving it as fuel more efficiently.

If you already love eating real foods, I'm not telling you to go out and buy a bunch of processed junk. That's reversing your progress, and we're not here to backslide. But if you're hooked on these processed junk foods, try to buy less of them and wean yourself off over time.

If at the beginning of your low carb plan you just can't give up bread, maybe eat a sandwich with only one slice of bread every few days. You'll want to work on giving bread and other highly processed carbs up completely, but at the beginning you may need that bread to make it through the day. That one piece of bread one or two times each week may be the key factor in helping you stay committed long term.

I basically grew up eating processed foods, and even when I tried to lose weight with 'healthy' diets, the plans I encountered were mostly filled with more processed foods.

When I tried to go all in with low carb plans and attempted to give up all of my favorite processed foods in the past, I failed miserably. When I allowed my body time to wean off my favorite junk foods, that's when I found success.

Of course, I also kept track of carbs while weaning off the junk, so this isn't a free for all just because you're addicted to carbs. You need to go into this method with the intentions that you'll eat less and less of these foods each week, until you eventually eat mostly real food that your body knows how to process.

This means you'll eat more real food and less processed food whenever you have the choice. Save those junky processed foods for a time your body is really crying out for them. When this happens, be sure to add what you plan to eat to your plate, and don't eat more than maybe half of a serving listed on the package. Give yourself a little taste, but don't go overboard.

Once you start eating, it may be hard to stop because your brain remembers how easy it is to pull energy from these foods. Your goal here is to stop at just a little bit. You'll also be making better choices with protein and healthy fats with each meal, so you won't end up feeling overly hungry by just sticking with a little bit of your favorite foods.

If you're unable to stop at half of a serving, then maybe it's time to take these foods out completely. While this is the harder route, continuing to binge on foods filled with carbs won't push you towards your goal.

Stop Screaming Squirrel!

Another huge tip to transitioning to a keto lifestyle long term is to quit starting diet after diet. You need to choose your path and stick with it. If at some point you fall off that path, do the next right thing. Get right back on your plan instead of beating yourself up about it. Doing the next right thing is the only way you'll see long term progress.

Berating yourself because you fell off your plan will only cause mental damage that will make it harder to find long term success. Losing weight is more than just what you eat and how much you exercise. There's a huge mental component to weight loss, and you have to teach yourself to master that mental component.

Quit feeling bad about yourself because of a diet slip up. Follow the path you choose as closely as you can. If you fall off, get right back on. This will save you a lot of frustration and failed attempts.

I know from experience how dieters start a diet on Monday and do very well with it, at least until Friday. Then you become overwhelmed by your physiology and give into cravings. All of the sudden the weekend becomes a free for all. You eat every piece of junk you can shove into your face, right before you vow to start again on Monday.

If this is you, raise your hand. Now slap yourself in the head with that raised hand, and vow to quit following this pattern.

Seriously, don't do this. This is never the way to make it to your ultimate goal of thinner thighs and better health. This self destructive behavior is keeping you stuck in diet mentality, and it's making life way harder than it needs to be.

It also means your physiology is out of whack, and you need to take steps to actively help your body process the food you eat better. And no, that big smack to your head wasn't enough to knock your physiology back into balance.

You need to take the steps to improve how your body digests the food you should be eating. This includes real food that's filled with healthy fats and protein.

Not everyone needs to take this step, but if you've jumped from diet to diet over the years, or if you've previously tried low carb and struggled to stick with it, you will need to take this step.

Also, if you've had poor health for many years, and you've relied on your fair share of medications to make it through the day, it's time to learn how improving digestion can make these changes both more effective and easier.

You can learn more about which supplements to take in order to work with your body to make this all easier in that digestion course I mentioned earlier. I can't tell you exactly what you need in this book because *A. I'm not a doctor* and *B. everyone is different and our different chemistries require different approaches.* Putting in the effort to research your own health is 100% worth your time.

To be honest, low carb never worked for me before I took steps to improve digestion. I honestly don't believe it ever would have worked without this step.

While giving my body time to adjust by lowering carbs and making swaps from processed food to real food over time would have resulted in some progress, I never would have made it to my ultimate goal, nor would I have seen such drastic health improvements, without following the improved digestion piece.

A Different Approach

So why am I advising you to do this all slowly when so many other health experts want you to rip off the bandaid and jump straight into their nicely laid out plan?

I think part of it is I tried that approach for years, and it never worked for me. It was too extreme of an approach, and I never allowed my body time to adjust. I expected to burn glucose one day and fat the next. Unfortunately, it's never that easy for most people.

Many of the health experts who tell you to rip off the bandaid and dive headfirst into these plans took up residence in the health field because they've had health issues of their own at some point. Now that they've resolved their issues, they can tell you how to follow a proper keto diet, or even how to fast for best results, but most of what they teach isn't exactly how they started.

Perhaps they have good intentions, and they want you to skip past their mistakes. While that's an honorable notion, the truth is, they allowed their bodies ample time to adjust while making those mistakes. Their physiology had time to improve.

Most of these experts didn't jump straight from the standard American diet one day, into a strict keto plan the next where they ate less than 20 carbs and noshed on way more fat than they could effectively digest.

These experts had time to adjust while going through trial and error. Telling you to jump straight into a strict keto plan before you're ready can be a recipe for disaster for many.

The same thing is true for fasting.

If an expert tells you that following OMAD works for him now, and that's the solution to everyone's problems because it worked for him, don't follow that expert. No one thing will ever be right for everyone.

Sure, OMAD, which stands for one meal a day, may work for some people for weight loss, but it will actually slow a lot of people down.

You need to consider if that expert started out on an OMAD plan, or did he start with a different fasting plan, and then eventually ended up on OMAD once he already found success with a different method?

Intermittent fasting is a little more advanced than we're talking about in this chapter, but I wanted to use that example because I've seen others start out on an OMAD plan since some expert used different fasting plans to lose weight, and then stuck with OMAD for maintenance. Now everyone who follows this expert thinks they should jump right into what's working for him now.

Whether you follow a low carb, keto or even an intermittent fasting plan, you need to follow the plan that's right for you and right for your physiology - where you are now. Quit trying to force a plan you're not ready for just because it worked for someone else; or it's working now for someone else after he had a trial and error time period to adjust.

If you keep starting a keto plan that's 20 carbs per day, but you always fall off the keto wagon, it's time to reassess. It's time to look at your physiology and determine what you can do differently to find low carb success over the long term, instead of another quick fix you pray will work this time around.

I feel like I'm getting preachy, and I definitely don't want to be preachy.

Let's sum up the easy tricks you can do right now to build a low carb a lifestyle that will work for you if you're coming from the standard American diet, or if you've attempted low carb, but you can't seem to stick with it long term:

1. Start by lowering your carbs to 25 grams of carbs or less per meal.

2. Once you have that part down, take it a little bit further and lower carbs even more at one of those meals to 15 carbs or less … so either breakfast or dinner will be under 15 grams of carbs, and your other two meals will be closer to 20 or 25 grams of carbs.

3. If you include snacks, keep the carbs in those snacks very low. Be sure to pair any carbs you do eat with healthy fats so the insulin spike is lower.

4. If you can eat lower to medium glycemic foods at snacks and meals do this, otherwise transition to this overtime if you're not ready.

5. Take the time to look at how you're digesting the foods you should focus on eating, like healthy fats and proteins.

   a. If you show signs of not digesting these foods well, taking the steps to improve this will make this lifestyle so much easier, especially when it comes to long term results.

b. If you experience symptoms like constipation, diarrhea, acne, gas, bloating, heartburn, the list can go on and on; but if you experience these kinds of health issues, it's time to take steps to improve this so you can find low carb success long term.

6. Don't jump right into keto if your body isn't ready for it since you can still see success with low carb. While it may be slower success, trying to force keto when you're not ready likely means you won't see long term success anyway, so quit trying to force it if you haven't improved digestion, or if you haven't given your body time to adjust to your new fuel source.

Chapter 3: A.C. 1 - Living the Low-carb Life

If you read *My Big Fat Life Transformation*, heard my story in an interview, or even if you've participated in any of my courses, one thing you've heard me mention is how I lost at least 70 pounds before I even knew what a ketogenic diet was.

I sometimes talk in general phrases like "at least" or "somewhere around," because I honestly don't have exact numbers of what I lost, and during which phase I lost it.

I've been stuck in this dieting world for so long where I was constantly in a cycle of weight loss, followed by weight regain, that I honestly never expected to hit my goal with any plan. I definitely never dreamed I'd dip below my goal weight and stay there with ease for more than three years. I for sure never expected to teach what I learned to anyone who wanted to listen.

I like to look at my story as three phases, where each phase was an important stepping stone into the next. Each phase helped me take what I'd normally consider just another diet I was following, and helped me solidify low carb and keto as a lifestyle.

In the last chapter I talked about the steps you can take to transition from the standard American diet to a low carb plan. If you're already further down the line, you may be OK to skip this chapter. It's a long one, but it really digs into the steps for those who just can't seem to stay on track with any low carb plan longer than a few days at a time.

For everyone else, let me show you the steps I took in more detail that helped solidify my low carb diet into a plan I stuck to long term. This was an important step for me in order to turn keto into my permanent lifestyle.

When you adjust your mindset from just another diet to your new lifestyle, that's when this all becomes easy and magical. That's when you no longer struggle each day to make it through a life you hate, hoping to find a life you'll eventually love, but only once you hit your goal weight.

Now if you're thinking, "Cool - if referring to keto as my lifestyle instead of calling it a diet will melt the pounds away, sign me up!" Um yeah, it doesn't really work that way. Don't ask me how I know.

OK, so I'll admit I've also heard this lecture many times before. I thought if I could force a mindset switch to view low carb as my lifestyle, then poof! My goal weight would be within reach. Some people make you believe it can be that simple, even though we all know it's never that simple.

When I was still in that dieting cycle where I desperately attempted diet after diet in order to find a plan that finally worked for me, I remember this one particular day when I was out for a walk with my dog, Wrigley.

During the walk, I repeated several mantras to myself like, "This is my new lifestyle. I will lose all of the weight I want to lose. I will remain at my goal weight this time. I will love the (likely disgusting) diet food I eat, and I will never crave processed junk again."

I thought repeating these statements over and over was the way I could cement a new lifestyle into my brain once and for all. Wrigley got a chance to poop, and I practiced drilling my new mindset into my brain. That's what I like to call multitasking.

I honestly thought if I could force a mindset change, maybe I'd finally hit my goal weight, and somehow magically stay there forever. Change your mind, change your life, right?

Is it necessary to have a positive mindset? Yes.

Is it great to repeat mantras to yourself every day until you reach your goal? Yes.

Is it helpful to envision yourself at your goal weight before you get there? Yes.

Do I feel like I'm talking in a condescending manner like Kate Gosselin by asking questions I plan to answer myself? Yes.

I'll stop that now.

My point with all of these questions is that all of these wonderful approaches *can* help you along your weightloss journey. I did all of these things on my journey to lose more than 100 pounds, and they all helped me gain momentum towards my ultimate destination.

But is making this mindshift the only step I had to take to reach my ultimate goal?

OK, I really need to stop asking questions I plan to answer. I'm starting to feel the urge to get a weird a-line haircut chopped to the top of my left ear. If I really was just like *Kate plus 8*, I'd condescendingly guilt you into diet compliance, and you would listen because that chick is scary.

We should all be deathly afraid of any woman who would dare go out in public with a big spiky poof on the top of her head. I'm pretty sure that hairstyle was used in a secret weapon of some sort. That's the *only* explanation as to why Jon Gosselin went into hiding in his hometown of Wyomissing, Pennsylvania.

Seriously, he lives in a town called Wyo-missing. Look it up.

OK, I know we're still getting to know each other, but I swear I'm not scary like that mean mugging mom of eight. Also, I know entirely way too much about Jon and Kate Gosselin for never having watched an episode of *Jon and Kate plus 8*.

My computer also somehow knows way too much since autocorrect automatically changed the spelling from J-o-h-n to J-o-n.

But my answer is no; not even close!

Attempting to force a mindset change and telling myself all of the things I wanted to happen didn't automatically make them happen. There was still a whole lotta work I had to put into my plan to make the progress I wanted to make.

While all of this mindset and positivity stuff is important to stay motivated long term, especially if you have a lot of weight to lose like I did, forcing a mindset change like this won't make you the next low carb success story. You still need to put in the work to turn low carb into your new lifestyle.

This means eating foods that are right for your physiology, while also taking any necessary steps you need to in order to improve digestion. We've talked about all of this countless times by now, right? But have you taken the time to figure out what this means for you?

I know you're already committed to keto, and that seems like a lot of change all at once. I know asking you to test your body chemistry seems like adding even more work, and ain't nobody got time for that.

The only reason I keep talking about this is because following these steps can lead to long term results that actually stick. Finding foods that are right for your chemistry right now, and then changing them as your body chemistry changes along the way, can make it like you're cheating on your diet … but in a good way.

When you learn how to work with your body instead of following random advice you find that worked for someone else, this makes you a cheater who wins! While cheaters who win are rare, this is one of the few times you can cheat for better results, and actually feel good about your big ole' cheatin' self.

If I got you all hyped up about cheating your way to better results, you can start the digestion course here. For only 50 cents, you'll learn how to start working with your body instead of forcing changes that aren't right for you, right now.

And that 50 cents you'll spend ain't making anybody rich, mmmkay? So you better believe I keep linking that course in this book since you probably need this help to get unstuck from yo-yo plans forever!

It's Just A Phase

For keto to eventually become my lifestyle, I went through three different phases. These include a low carb phase where I lowered carbs to approximately 25 grams per meal, while also taking time to improve chemistry imbalances and digestion; followed by a keto phase, where I lowered carbs to only 20-30 total grams each day; and finally a more strict keto and IF phase where I added daily intermittent fasting to the mix.

This chapter is all about that first phase I went through that helped establish low carb as my new way of eating. Many other keto experts nudge you to jump head first into the deep end. They urge a strict keto plan of less than 20 carbs from the start, while also eating more fat than your body knows what to do with.

I personally believe if I never took the time to hang out in this low carb phase for at least a little while, I never would have found success with keto long term. In fact, I can say that with 100% confidence because I've tried keto type diets in the past, and I failed 100% of the time.

After my first pregnancy, I attempted to return to over-exercise and low calorie plans in order to lose the extra hundred pounds or so that I un-willingly had mashed onto my body. Since expectations to lose 100 pounds were daunting and seemed downright impossible, I never established that big number as my ultimate goal.

I went into weight loss this time around with a goal of getting out of the XXL maternity clothes I wore during pregnancy. I would have given anything just to get back into the size 14 Torrid jeans I dreaded wearing pre-pregnancy.

In fact, I never put a number on the amount of weight I wanted to lose at all. Sure, losing more than 100 pounds would have been the goal for my twenty-something self, but I was over thirty and a busy mom. I had to be practical.

Basically, not in the 200's would have been perfectly suitable for me. Never did I ever think I'd make it to such a hopeless place in my dieting life that I'd actually be ecstatic to weigh 199 pounds. But I was in such a low place when it came to dieting, that even getting out of the 200's, a place I'd never previously been, seemed unlikely.

Around six months post pregnancy, I determined cutting calories no longer worked for me. Despite my best efforts, I continually lost and regained the same three to five pounds. Exercising on my gym quality elliptical even harder, while cutting calories even lower, did nothing. I spent many nights in tears because I thought all of the yo-yo dieting I did over the past few decades broke my metabolism. I truly believed I was stuck at this higher weight for life. In my mind, I was destined for a life of oversized mom jeans paired with XXL flowy tops that only came in ugly floral patterns.

Seriously, can't us bigger girls get a little more variety without spending our life's savings on a shirt to hide our excess fluff?

Listen, I know I wear medium tops these days, but I was in and out of larger sizes for most of my life. Most women who follow this type of trend will always identify as a bigger girl, no matter her current size. Please don't accuse me of plus sized cultural appropriation.

The Book That Changed My Life

With the calories in versus calories out method failing me big time, I was desperate for a new solution. I continued to read every diet book I could find on Amazon. Some friends on social media talked about a book called *The Diet Game*. It's a book where you compete against others to lose weight. I thought maybe that was the kick in the butt I needed to finally get the pounds off.

I went directly to Amazon to purchase the book that would surely change my life forever.

While I was there, another book called *Kick Your Fat in the Nuts* was advertised as free, so I thought sure, why not get that book too to save for a rainy day. I lived in Chicago at the time, and we had plenty of rainy days, which meant I read plenty of well meaning diet books.

I devoured *The Diet Game*, which talked about competing as a group to lose weight. There were suggested steps in the book to help with weight loss. Of course, I could follow those steps on my own, but I really wanted to participate with a group to help with motivation.

I sought out to join the diet game group of the girl who I saw talking about the book. I kind of knew her from high school, although I don't remember us being friends.

Somehow we reconnected through Facebook and saw each other's posts. That was really the extent of our friendship. I was desperate to lose the baby weight, and she also just had a baby - so I thought it would be great to have a buddy who was in the same place in life. I asked to join her group.

While she was super nice about my request, she let me know her game was already filled and they were in the middle of a competition. She told me she'd let me know as soon as the next game opened up.

I understood, yet was disappointed since no dieter on a mission to shed pounds wants to wait until the next game. If there's a Monday on the horizon that isn't a holiday, us dieters are determined to begin our new diets, come hell or high water.

I printed the game materials and tried to get my husband on board, but I don't think he was really into it. I posted my results on the fridge hoping he'd see this magical new plan I was following, and eventually he'd join. I'm sure he just figured this was the latest and greatest diet scam I was following, and he didn't think it would last long enough for him to get involved.

Truth is, I only made it through about a month of the diet game before it had too many rules to follow. Then, I was onto the next plan.

This brings me back to that other book I found on Amazon that day that actually did change my life - *Kick Your Fat in the Nuts.*

A few pages into the book, after learning it was written by a comedian, I was sold! Who doesn't love comedic diet plans? Satan! That's who.

I actually did come across a girl, who may or may not be a stick-in-the-mud family member who surely will never read this book with a slight humorous edge, and she told me she couldn't get through the book because of the jokes.

Um, say what now?

Do you not like to enjoy this daily grind we call life? Do you not wish to find humor in something as mind numbing and challenging as losing excess weight that seems to be clinging onto your body for dear life?

Looking back, she's one of those people who finds joy in chronic complaining about her daily grind, so it makes sense. She always seems to have a new ailment that's ruining her day, and she's ready to cry about it to anyone who will show compassion.

Ironically enough, many of the ailments she complains of are addressed in the book. If she only buckled down for all of those jokes that ruined her day, she could've found real solutions to her ailments. Sadly there are some people out there who just like to be sick, and snide remarks about a diet industry that fails us over and over can never change that.

Back to me.

So while I'd previously never actually tried a comedic diet plan, I was a huge fan of VH1's *Stand-Up Spotlight* back in the day, so I was sold! Sad, chronic complainer I am not! Enjoyer of all the humor life has to offer - sign me up.

I was ready to laugh, learn and lose all the weight! Then reality hit.

A few pages in I realized this was not a comedic diet plan at all. I realized I was reading yet another book that talked about using a low carb plan to lose weight. My. Heart. Sank.

Much of the information I read in this book was new, and seemed to be the fresh start I needed. I really wanted to follow through on this plan that seemed too good to be true, but I started and failed so many low carb plans in the past that I wanted no part of another low carb diet.

I was finally cool with eating low calorie as long as I could eat bread. I was even ok with gnawing hunger while constantly feeling weak while losing weight, but I was done with giving up crunchy chips forever. Low carb was no longer in the cards for me. I'd been there, done that and declared myself done with nixing my favorite foods forever. I was ready for a more sensible plan I could actually stick to this time. I was ready for a plan I could follow forever.

Sure, previously I had some success dropping weight with low carb, but I always felt awful during the process. I dreaded low carb diets because I missed occasional junk food like a side of fries, or a dinner roll with butter. It pained me mentally to think about giving up my favorites again in what would likely result as another failed low carb attempt.

How long would I even last this time around? It all seemed so pointless.

Still, I was desperate to take off this weight that would not budge via any other method in my weight loss arsenal. The book also promised I'd fix up some other health ailments that plagued me for the majority of my life.

Thanks comedic author sir, because that part gave me a good laugh. These problems I dealt with were hereditary - we all know this.

How would changing my diet fix genes I can't control being born with? Genes that led to chronic ailments, such as daily headaches and constant anxiety. Needless to say, I'd been given so many similar promises throughout my life that I wasn't buying the health wisdom this book was selling. At least not all of it.

I decided to follow the steps in the book, but I was really only in it for the weight loss. I never bought into the false hope that I'd improve health problems that had become my BFF's over the past 20 years.

Seriously, if daily headaches, monthly sinus infections, cystic acne and anxiety all could have worn the other half of one of those BFF heart necklaces, they'd have to fight it out for which symptom would have gotten to wear the other half of my broken heart necklace. I had many health ailment BFF's to go around, all fighting to be my one true bestie for life.

I did order the supplements suggested, which include Beet Flow, Beatine HCL, Digestizyme and Bio C. While it says very clearly in the book that these are not magical weight loss supplements, in my diet obsessed mind I was only taking them for the weight loss aspect.

While I didn't understand all of the nuances of the supplement routine at the time, if people shot these down the hatch, and that led to busting through weight loss plateaus, I didn't really care about the backstory or how they worked - I was taking those pills!

Poof! Baby weight, be gone!

When I began the supplement routine as suggested, and I performed the chemistry tests I didn't quite understand, I also began changing the food I put into my body to go along with the strategy the book promotes. Although the book does talk a lot about eating low-to-medium glycemic index carbs with meals that should be around 25 grams of carbs per meal, that's not the route I took at the beginning. To me, a carb was a carb was a carb, and the fact that I was lowering carbs at all was a huge battle I was still fighting with myself.

I acquiesced to most meals around 25 grams of carbs, but I was stubborn and still did it my way. After all, I spent the previous twenty years devouring every diet article and book I came across, so I knew best, right?

This girl who was constantly losing and regaining the same 20 to 50 pounds surely knew everything there was to know about losing weight, right?

Yeah, not so much.

I knew a ton, but that ton was the info the mainstream wanted me to know. What they wanted me to know was all of the wrong information to keep me coming back for more of what this 88 billion dollar diet industry had to offer. Not that everyone is bad and out to get us, but there's just enough wrong information put out to keep us confused.

This bad info spreads like wildfire, and you end up considering it an absolute truth. This keeps you confused and stuck. Now you no longer know how to discern the good info from the bad, and you ultimately end up blaming yourself when you fail. That's a drama for another day since today we're talking about how I finally finagled my body to stick with a low carb plan for good.

A Day In The low carb Life

So like Old Blue Eyes, I did it my way.

I ate 25 carbs with each meal, but nary a sweet potato passed through my lips. The 25 carbs I ate with meals at the start included maybe eating only one slice of bread with my sandwich instead of two. If I had enough carbs leftover for the meal, I'd also add half a serving of potato chips, because this girl had a major addiction to those crunchy slices of potatoey heaven.

My husband and I still ate many meals out each week, so I typically ordered a lot of burgers and removed the buns. That's just *low carb 101.*

Except I really loved the buns, so at first I'd still eat at least a few bites of each bun with my meal. I also added a small handful of fries. This way it still felt like I was eating one of my favorite meals, but I wasn't completely filling myself up on every last bite of the junk like I had in the past.

Low Carb Breakfast

For breakfast, I'd typically keep a meal as low in carbs as possible. I always seemed to feel better and have a better chance at keeping the rest of my day on track when I had a really good start to the day.

I never really loved eggs growing up, but as with many low carb diets in the past, I added them back in as many days as I could because they're an easy low carb breakfast that seemed to keep me fuller longer. I also added in a few pieces of breakfast sausage, and topped everything with butter to make it all taste better.

My blood pressure was very low, so I topped it all off with a high quality sea salt to complete the meal. The only thing I really left out was the whole wheat toast I previously enjoyed. Sure, I still loved bread topped with butter as much as the next girl, but I really wanted to lose weight, so it was a sacrifice I was willing to make.

On days I really missed carbs, I'd add in a few slices of a lower carb fruit, like cantaloupe or a few strawberries. I had a food scale at home, so I was sure to measure out only the amount of carbs I wanted to add to breakfast. I didn't make a habit of this everyday since I tried to keep breakfast as low in carbs as possible.

Also, per the book's suggestion, I added a coconut yummy after each meal to help my body learn to love coconut oil, because at first, I didn't really love the taste. It wasn't a taste that necessarily made me gag, but it also wasn't something I'd have chosen voluntarily.

On the days I didn't want eggs, I'd make a protein shake instead. I found a high quality protein mix that was lower in carbs. I read in the book that liquid carbs were public enemy #1, so it was important to really dig into that label and make sure I found a protein mix that was lower in carbs.

I started out simple by adding almond milk, a touch of melted coconut oil and the protein mix. Over time I wanted to add more healthy components to my daily shake, while cutting carbs even lower, so eventually I swapped almond milk for water and I began adding handfuls of spinach to the shakes. I gradually added more coconut oil as my body was better able to digest fat.

Looking back, I'd probably also skip the water and make my shake with heavy cream instead. Even then, I was still all about the calories, and heavy cream is heavy on calories. It took me years into my low carb plan to learn the calorie lessons I needed to learn, and now teach to anyone who'll listen.

When I was really ready to make it the healthiest shake I could, I cut the protein mix in half, which cut liquid carbs even more, and I added in a high quality collagen protein instead.

I also began chopping up more green food, like cucumbers, to add to the shake. While adding spinach had minimal impact on taste, adding cucumbers definitely made for a different taste, and not necessarily in a good way. It was eventually a taste my body became accustomed to, and eventually craved.

This is how a lot of my current eating habits came to be. I made small, gradual adjustments over time to help my body begin to prefer the healthier substitutions over time. Of course, I didn't realize the impact these adjustments would have on my life since I didn't go into this plan with the intentions of keeping these habits around forever.

Slowly shifting from bad, to ok, to a little better, to good, to "Wow, that's super healthy!" was the best way for me to transition over time. This process eventually made, "Wow that's super healthy!" into the way I lived life most of the time.

This shift didn't happen overnight, but the important point to note is that it happened.
Instead of forcing changes my body wasn't ready for in order to lose weight as quickly as possible, I allowed changes to happen gradually. My body rewarded me with the ability to more easily stick to these changes long term. This means I get to enjoy the health benefits long term instead of constantly tracking down the latest quick fix fad.

With this gradual shift, I was finally free of the yo-yo diet pattern that plagued me for decades. This was something I never previously thought possible. I honestly believed I'd struggle with my weight for as long as I cared, until one day I settled into a life lived in flowy muumuus and fuzzy slippers.

I'm being serious here. I even planned to create my own line of fancy muumuus to sell on the high end market. Asa from *The Shahs of Sunset* beat me to it; she just calls them kaftans.

Looking back, I'm glad I didn't follow through with these #lifegoals since I never really stood a chance against her. Chick had a show on Bravo, plus all of that Jackson family money to help her out.

Low Carb Lunch

Now that we covered my typical breakfast, let's talk lunch.

Around the noon hour, I ate a lot of sandwiches with only one piece of bread when I first began low carb. Once I felt ready, I gave up bread entirely and ate rolled up lunch meat with all of the fixings.

I stuck with half servings of chips as a side a lot of the time. Some days I was 'healthy' and ate an apple dipped in peanut butter instead of chips. Apples are fruit, so that makes apples a good choice, right?

Yes, an apple is a far better choice than processed potato chips and taking steps in the direction of replacing processed foods with real food like that turned out to be great choices for my lifestyle over time. However, eating apples on your low carb plan isn't something I'd recommend long term; at least not when you're aiming for weight loss.

If you need these types of higher sugar foods to transition to your next phase like I did, by all means, eat an apple instead of overly processed foods like potato chips. At the same time, please realize just because an apple is a real food, and real food is what we should eat, this doesn't make an apple an appropriate choice for everyone.

Apples are high in sugar, which means they can cause a greater insulin spike for many. This insulin spike may be too high for some to see progress, especially when they start adding in as much fat as a keto diet requires.

If you love apples, I'd recommend eating only half, adding some fat to keep your insulin spike lower, and only using apples as a stepping stone to get to the next level of your low carb plan. Apples will always be there for you to test bringing back in once you reach your goal.

Low Carb Snacks

For snacks, I did my best to keep them under 15 grams of carbs. I typically ate one or two snacks each day, depending on hunger. I was still a slave to processed convenience foods, so I ate a lot of 'healthy' bars that claimed to be lower in carbs on the package. I still went by net carbs, so I ate bars that were using artificial sweeteners and weird fibers.

I knew from previous experience that living on these processed convenience foods as meals did nothing for my progress, so I didn't use these as meals. I ate them as snacks whenever I had a craving for something like that.

I did try, whenever possible, to eat more real food snacks like nuts, seeds and cheese. I'd also chop up cucumbers and dip them in ranch dressing as a snack. I'm a creature of habit when it comes to food, so I pretty much rotated these snacks and ate whatever I was in the mood for that day.

Low Carb Dinner

For dinners, I made a lot of the same meals because I wasn't really a great cook. I knew how to cook spaghetti sauce with meat, so I found a low sugar marinara sauce I liked and used that. I chopped up the veggies I enjoyed, like green peppers and onions, and added those to the sauce. I added ground beef too, but these were all of the same steps I used before low carb to make spaghetti sauce. The only difference was I sought out a low sugar sauce.

I also still added noodles at the beginning of my low carb plan. Instead of grabbing a big heap of noodles like I was used to, I'd measure out only half of a serving of pasta and topped it with plenty of meat sauce in order to stay satiated. The next time I made spaghetti, I used less noodles, and continued with that pattern until I no longer needed noodles at all.

This was the same pattern I followed with most meals. I was coming from the standard American diet, where many people eat up to 300 grams of carbs each day, so eating only 75 - 150 carbs daily made a huge difference, even if I didn't jump right into the deep end with eating only real food carbs like berries and sweet potatoes.

I'll be honest - after a lifetime of processed foods that were artificially sweetened, I didn't enjoy the taste of sweet potatoes or berries. If I forced these changes before my body was ready, I don't think they would have lasted very long, and I'd be stuck in the world of yo-yo diets to this day. I'd still be trying to figure out how to lose weight, while existing on foods made in a lab instead of slowly learning how to eat the real foods my body was designed to consume.

Today I love sweet potatoes and berries ... but that love of real food took time for me to develop. I also love broccoli, zucchini and spinach. Never did I ever think I would make such a bold proclamation.

Brussel sprouts ... meh. I still can't get behind the round chunks of stinky green that are brussel sprouts. My husband loves brussel sprouts, and orders them often. Everytime he does, my 4 year old says, "Dad, what do you say?" since, let's be honest - brussel sprouts carry the same aroma as most men's lingering farts.

Other Important Changes

Most people add some kind of dessert or late night snack after dinner. Even though I wasn't following 100% of the rules as I should have right away, I still knew I was on a diet with weight loss as the goal, so I cut out after dinner snacking entirely.

Sure it was tough for this girl who loved to eat an entire bag of microwave popcorn every night while undwinding with her favorite shows, but after just a few nights of getting out of this bad habit, the good habit of not snacking after dinner became easy.

This was when I began intermittent fasting light. What I mean by this is I would go 12 hours in between my last bite of dinner, and before my first bite of breakfast. While this used to just be normal, and some people fall into this pattern naturally, let's be honest - most people pop food into their mouths from the second they open their eyes until right before their heads hit the pillow at night. Going 12 hours without food can be challenging for many, myself included.

I stuck with it, and eventually this too became a habit.

As the year went on, I continued to improve food choices. I dropped the high glycemic index carbs like pasta and bread all together, and began to favor more real food options instead. I still kept many meals around 25 carbs per meal, except breakfast, which was commonly even lower. All of the carbs I did eat provided a lower insulin spike than the 25 grams of bread carbs I ate at the beginning, so I made a lot of progress over time.

The gradual improvements resulted in big changes over the course of a year. Not only did I finally get out of that cycle I was stuck in for more than six months of losing and regaining the same three to five pounds over and over, but my weight kept going lower and lower.

Sure, it wasn't the dramatic five pound weight loss every week that every dieter secretly desires, but I was consistent at losing weight most weeks. Some weeks it was two pounds, while others it may have been only half of a pound. There were even some weeks the scale went up a little. Over time the losses outweighed any small gains I had, and those small losses added up to a big loss of 70 pounds that first year alone.

Benefits Beyond Weight Loss

Not only was I 70 pounds lighter, but my fasting blood sugars, which were in diabetic ranges when I began, completely normalized after only a few months. I noticed I was no longer getting monthly sinus infections, and my daily headaches were much less frequent. Many of the other health problems I dealt with for decades were either drastically improved, or simply vanished.

I went into that first year of lowering carbs and taking steps to improve my chemistry and digestion with a goal of getting out of the 200's. Here I was, one year later, around 170 pounds. I was finally back into the size 14 jeans I was so desperate to wear. In fact, those jeans fit loosely, and I felt so much healthier.

I never thought I'd get rid of years of embarrassing and painful acne, but I did.

I never thought I'd go years without experiencing migraines so bad that I'd have to lay down in a dark room for the day, but they're gone.

I never thought I'd be done with yo-yo diets where I constantly lost and regained every single pound, but I am.

And I did it my way.

Well, not really my way. My way would have been filled with all the bread and processed junk foods I loved, while somehow still magically shedding fat. While I did go into low carb kicking and screaming this time around, I tried it my way for decades and I never found the success I wanted.

I didn't love the idea of starting another low carb diet, but I'm so happy I trusted what I learned this time around. I'm thankful I didn't jump head first into restricting all of the carbs right away, or I didn't immediately convert to all real foods all of the time, no matter how much my mind resisted.

I tried those methods, and they weren't right for me. Instead, I took my time, weaned myself from the junk, and used the supplements to give my body that extra push it needed to function properly.

I know at times some of this info may seem repetitive throughout the book. A lot of dieters have been brainwashed, and it takes a lot of repetition for the right information to sink in. Trust me, I was brainwashed for more than two decades!

Highlight the points that seem too crazy to be true. Go back and read them again since they're probably the very points that will help you escape the diet roller coaster forever!

If you're reading this chapter for the therapy session, or perhaps looking to laugh at yet another embarrassing story of my diet trials and tribulations, but you're more advanced than 25 carbs per meal, I'm not advising you to backslide if you're already on your merry keto way.

If your daily diet already consists of real food that is low in carbs, and you're not struggling to get these foods onto your plate everyday, this chapter is not advising you to add back the junk.

If you're coming from a similar place as I did where low carb never seems to stick, I want you to know there's hope for you. I want you to know that it doesn't have to be all or nothing. All or nothing plans surely have failed you time and again in the past, just as they have for me.

It's OK to make small improvements and learn to love this low carb lifestyle gradually over time. It's OK to take baby steps if that's all you're ready to take right now. The important part is to continue to move forward on your path, even if the steps you take each day are small steps. Be sure that today is better than yesterday, and that tomorrow you vow to move forward another step.

If you look for continual, gradual improvements over time, you'll eventually reach your goal. If you jump head first into an all or nothing plan that your body isn't physiologically ready for, you're headed for the same fate you had last time you tried this same approach.

Chapter 4: Avoid Diet Obsession

This entire book is based on turning keto into your lifestyle. One of the most important obstacles you may face is learning to live a keto lifestyle without feeling the obsession most dieters have when they begin a new plan.

If you're new to keto, or even if you've followed keto for a while, but you still find yourself thinking about your diet more often than you should, there's a better way to convert to your new lifestyle.

There are so many new things to learn and incorporate when you first adopt a ketogenic lifestyle. First there's the macros and the macro percentages. Should you follow 75/15/10, or perhaps 85/10/5?

And what the heck do those numbers even mean?

Then there's food choices. Some people shove down anything labeled low carb, while others swear that processed foods with labels aren't keto legal. And don't forget about the sweeteners. Since many say a real food keto diet removes most artificial sweeteners, why can you only find keto recipes with tons of sweeteners added?

With so much new information to sort through and customize, there's pretty much no way to turn keto into your lifestyle without obsessing, am-I-right?

It's hard to adapt any diet as your new lifestyle without at least a little obsession. Now that so many new changes have been thrown at you all at once, how can you turn keto into your lifestyle without keto taking over your life?

If your feet have been firmly planted in the dieting world for some time, there's a high likelihood you've become obsessed over a diet at some point or another. Whether you admit it or not, there's a great chance that at some point you felt like your new diet has taken over your life. There may have even been times you felt like your new diet became the main focus of your life.

Since we all know that's not fun, and that obsessing over keto is no way to live your best life, let's talk about some simple changes you can make to turn keto into a lifestyle you love instead of a diet you endlessly obsess over. Let's make this an easy transition where you no longer feel the need to obsess.

I've been on both sides of the diet coin, so I can tell you first hand that constantly thinking about your next meal, or even the meal you desperately crave, but aren't allowing yourself, isn't a great way to live life.

As I may have mentioned once or twice by now, I tried low carb diets for decades and they never became my lifestyle. Not at least until I changed my mindset, and took some steps where low carb finally clicked. It wasn't until then that I took low carb from just another diet I was forcing upon myself and turned it into my lifestyle.

If you're still struggling turning a low carb, high fat diet into your lifestyle without becoming obsessive, I'm here to give you a big hug and confide that I was once you.

And by once, I mean that one time that lasted decades. I'm also here to let you know, keto life doesn't have to be as hard as you make it. There are more important things to focus on in life than food.

Let's work on making the food part easy so we can celebrate all of the other joys life has to offer - with our keto friendly party food, of course.

Before Keto Was A Thing

When I talk about the plans I tried out over my sordid yo-yo history, I usually refer to them as low carb. The reason for this is keto wasn't really a thing back then. Sure, it was invented in the early 1920's as an alternative treatment for epilepsy, but it definitely wasn't a diet that was popular for weight loss.

Low carb approaches for weight loss have been around at least since the *Dr. Atkins Diet Revolution* was first published in 1972. While I am approaching a milestone birthday many people reference as over the hill, I'm not old enough to have participated in the original Atkins plan, so low carb didn't become a thing for me until the Atkins Diet gained popularity again in the late 90's / early 2000's.

Technically, his new approach didn't become popular until 2003 when he released a new plan, but I like to think I'm always ahead of the diet curve since I remember first trying a low carb plan circa 1999. While following this plan, I definitely still rewarded myself with my favorite meal at Baker's Square, the Spicy Chicken Pita, at least once each week. That fluffy pita filled with spicy joy was absolute meal perfection.

The Spicy Chicken Pita was appropriately served in a shiny gold wrapper, which contained a thick pita stuffed with breaded chicken, melted swiss, red onions, tomatoes and ranch dressing. It also came with a heaping side of golden fries. While this obviously didn't fit my low carb plan, I always said no to pie.

Same, right?

I'll even admit that some weeks a Baker's Square visit may have happened more than once. While I could have opted for eggs or a salad, I always ordered the exact same meal each visit. Allow me to make an obvious point here - eating meals like that a few times each week, while lowering carbs and pumping up fat most other days, was bound to make me fatter. I only mention this because I know there are many of you reading this that follow keto in a similar pattern. You too are likely getting fatter.

If you're still following keto in this manner, I'm waving my hands frantically at you while yelling, "Stahp it Rahn!"

Just like Sammi & Ronnie's relationship on *Jersey Shore* was an obvious trainwreck that would never work, neither will this keto plan where you eat some very low carb meals with higher fat, mixed with meals that are made up of all the carbs, but are also high in fat.

Even if you're just sneaking in one or two of these meals on the weekend, you're headed for a Ronpage. He's got mugshots now, so it's probably not the best path to follow.

For those who still aren't caught up on *Jersey Shore*, what I'm saying here is this method won't work. You could maybe, possibly get some results if you follow a low carb plan, and you have a cheat meal like this every so often; but it's definitely not something I'd recommend on a regular basis.

For those of you who think you can just ditch the pita and fries in that meal, please understand that breaded chicken isn't low carb. If you find a Baker's Square still generous enough to make this meal, you'd have to ask for grilled chicken, no pita and no fries to make this meal more keto friendly.

I know this is *low carb 101* to many, but I still feel the need to spell it out because I've known people who tell me they're following a keto plan, and then I see them eating chicken that's been breaded and fried - and I don't mean in almond flour and coconut oil either.

I'm watching you eat your fried chicken and yelling, "Stahp it Rahn!" in my head because that's definitely not keto!

How Not To Attempt A Low Carb Plan

Let's focus back on my early low carb attempts.

I made my first real go at a low carb diet when the plan became popular in 2003. While I never talked about dieting much with others since for some strange reason I felt like dieting was a topic that should be kept secret, I gave this diet a go with a few work friends. We commonly ate lunch at restaurants like Bennigan's, where we ordered bunless burgers with side salads. We all had spectacular results; for a few weeks, anyway.

I have to be honest - when I first began dipping my toe into low carb, I had no idea how to cook. Sure, I'd sometimes call my mom and ask her *yet again* the baking temperature for chicken, but that's the end of the cooking knowledge I sought from my mom.

Mom's infamous casseroles, where she threw any and all leftover ingredients from the fridge into a new meal for a surprise dinner, was the reason I grew up eating a lot of fast food. Let's just say I never understood why people longed for mom's home cooked meals when I only longed for a Big Mac meal with a large fry, plus an orange drink.

I can now look back and realize that depending on eating most meals out during the day, and meals made mostly of dry chicken breast for dinner because you lack basic cooking skills, makes keto a hard plan to follow long term.

Sure, some restaurants are catching on and it's becoming easier to get a delicious low carb meal out; but now that I've learned to cook so many delicious keto options, I actually prefer mom's home cooked meals.

Except, I'm the mom, because my mom's cooking - still a no-go.

It's great knowing the quality of the ingredients used, as well as the basic understanding of which ingredients are used. For instance, did you know if you order an omelette at IHOP, they add pancake batter to the eggs? Something seemingly as innocent as an omelette can kick you right out of ketosis, and you're none the wiser.

Samesies for Starbucks. If you order an iced coffee drink of some sort, some baristas dump sweetener right into your drink without your consent.

Feel violated yet?

Not only do I like knowing that I'm not sabotaging my plan like all of these restaurants seem so hellbent on doing, but I'd also like to toot my own horn a bit here. Some of the meal options I've come up with should be served at these restaurants I visit.

I'm ok with bragging just a little here since looking back at my pitiful low carb beginnings, I never would have imagined this would become a truth.

Of course if you're a member of the Keto Decoded Courses, surely you've already tested out some of these tasty meals first hand, so you know my bragging isn't without merit. If you're as pitiful in the kitchen as I was at the beginning, we have demonstration videos showing you how quick and easy these recipes are.

No more boring breasts! At least, not of the chicken variety.

Ah tangents … I seem to be the queen of tangents. Hopefully they're at least mildly entertaining tangents.

So I gave Atkins a good old college try more than once. Sometimes I tried a repackaged Atkins plan like Protein Power, or maybe even South Beach. I know those have variances in their plans, but they were all more plans where I had to rid myself of my beloved carbs.

Every single time I went into these plans with big dreams of low carb success. Once I hit my goal, I had big dreams of adding back all of my favorite foods at my new skinny weight. Somehow I magically planned to stay there once I got there, but I still required an abundance of french fries in my life at some point.

They always seemed like magical plans with three to five pounds coming off each week, at least for the first few weeks. I never understood why the weight melted off those first few weeks, but by the time I hit the second phase where I raised carbs a little, it slowed to only a pound or two per week; or sometimes stalled all together. I desperately wanted the magic back of my fat seemingly melting away.

Of course once the results on the scale stalled, it was difficult for me to stay motivated. Why the heck was I giving up some of my favorite meals filled with delicious buns and fries for a mere half pound loss on the scale each week?

None of this made sense to me, especially when I could go back to counting calories, enjoy the food I was eating and see the same, if not better, results.

When I say 'enjoy the food I was eating,' at this point I didn't look forward to much of what was on my plate like I do now. There are a few different reasons for this that we will quickly review. If you're struggling to enjoy all of the delicious food you get to eat on a low carb plan, you might learn why you're struggling.

My mind really loved to play tricks on me when I was trying out these low carb plans. I was all gung-ho for at least the first week, with that attitude sometimes even lasting a few weeks. The plan was even, dare I say, easy at the beginning. I got to eat as much food as I wanted, and I still saw the scale move.

Wahoo! Let's cut all the carbs!

Once my brain and my body started feeling deprived of carbs, I was back to constant thoughts like, "Why am I doing this to myself?" or "This can't be a healthy diet, can it?"

I began this cycle where I felt sorry for myself. In the back of my mind I knew eating all of this high fat food couldn't possibly be good for me.

The media was in my ear flashing these big low carb weight loss success stories, but then the next big news story was about how Dr. Atkins is trying to kill us all with his high fat plan. It was all so confusing. After the first few weeks on a low carb plan, I never really felt great, so I talked myself out of low carb again.

Same. Cycle. Every. Single. Time.

Then I was back to counting calories. My life was a constant struggle like this where I went back and forth between low carb diets and low-calorie diets for years. Once I was a few weeks into either plan, it was like I was a crazy person talking myself out of the diet because I felt so miserable. The grass was always greener on the other side of the diet spectrum, so I'd flip plans again because surely the other way was better.

This constant dieting led to an obsession where my life became so focussed on what I ate, or more likely, what I didn't allow myself to eat.

I never felt great either. All of the low calorie plans I switched back and forth to, combined with way more cardio than any person should endure, resulted in many health problems along the way.

I never connected the health problems I faced with the food I ate, or with too much exercise. I, like many others, assumed those were the health cards I was dealt, and all I needed was some over the counter drugs to fix myself up.

It All Goes Back to Digestion

Hopefully by now you understand low carb diets never stuck for me until I took steps to improve the way my body was digesting fats and proteins. I'm pretty sure I flat out said this at some point during the last chapter.

So many years of hopping from diet to diet, and then using medications to mask the health problems that resulted, caused aspects of my digestion to malfunction.

If you see yourself in any of this story - the constant failure to thrive on low carb plans, or constantly hopping from diet to diet because it's too hard to stick with any one plan long term, the first place I'd recommend you start is with digestion.

Improving the way my body digests the food I eat was the single most important step that helped cement low carb as a lifestyle for me. I never succeeded with low carb for more than a few months prior to taking these steps.

I have to be honest for a moment. I took the supplements suggested kind of as a hail Mary because nothing else was working to lose the stubborn baby weight. Since I've taken so many diet supplements in my day that did nothing, in the back of my mind I didn't really think these supplements would help me lose weight either.

Guess what - they didn't help me lose weight.
This makes sense since the supplements I took to improve
digestion *aren't* magical weight loss supplements.

There are no quick fix pills in existence that will help you
magically lose weight, while also improving health problems. If
you're still searching for these mythical pills, "Stahp it Rahn!"

I know I was still looking for pills like that, even after hearing
so many people tell me they don't exist. I'm serious here - they
don't exist. Well, maybe they exist if you're hanging out in the
Illuminati with Jay and Bey, but most of us don't have that type
of status.

Stand back Beehive, I'm kidding. Please don't attack me in full
force on social media. That's only a fun rumor that Queen Bey
is part of the Illuminati, or that the Illuminati even exists. If it
does exist, I'm not even sure the Illuminati elite have access to
magical pills that can help with weight loss and better health.

If they did, I'm sure Oprah's gotta be part of that group, yet
she still struggles with her weight from time to time. (Oprah, if
you're reading this, call me 'cause I've tried Weight Watchers
so. many. times. and there's a much better way!)

OK, Beehive, et. al, I'm backing away slowly from the Beyonce
and friends chit chat.

Let's get back to the less controversial digestion supplements.
I guess in a roundabout way Beet Flow and HCL did help with
weight loss. Once my bile was flowing properly, and my body
was able to break down protein in a more efficient manner,
low carb became easy for me for the first time.

When I began taking the supplements, I kind of, sort of understood what they did ... but I wasn't sure I noticed much of a difference for a long time. It wasn't until I noticed many other chronic symptoms I dealt with for many years just start disappearing that I really understood the value of these supplements.

Listen very closely to this part: I'm not saying you should run out and buy all of the supplements because they helped me with my program. It doesn't work that way. Also, I'm not a doctor, so remember not to take anything talked about in this book as medical advice.

I am saying if you commonly experience the symptoms that go along with poor digestion, it's important to improve those symptoms if you want to see long term success. You need to determine if you're dealing with these issues, and then you need to learn the information that will help balance your chemistry and improve your digestive situation.

We are all different. Following the plan I followed exactly may not get you the results you desire. You have different chemistry and your digestion is at a different place than mine was, so unlike so many other diet book authors attempt to do, I can't tell you the exact steps to take. You'll notice that the approach of following exact rules likely didn't work for you in the past anyway.

If you're trying to figure out what is right for you, check out full descriptions of the supplements I used here.

OK, another chapter, another tangent; but this one was an important tangent.

This supplement tangent does lead me to the important point I was trying to make with this story. Having digestion that is properly functioning can lead to success with a low carb plan, and also to less obsessing over low carb diets.

If your body is able to break down the fuel you give it properly, this means your brain will get the fuel it needs to function. If your brain has the proper fuel to function, then you'll naturally obsess less over your diet because your brain can now focus on other aspects of life instead of constantly trying to figure out how you're going to survive because it's not getting the fuel it knows how to run on efficiently.

So many people screw up their bodies with low calorie diets and medications to mask symptoms, that their bodies no longer understand how to efficiently break down fat as fuel. These previous low calorie dieters attempt to force an immediate switch from the standard American diet to keto. Their brains go crazy attempting to find ways to get the fuel it knows how to use. Eventually these people give in and end up completely blowing their keto plan.

Most blame themselves for cheating because carbs taste good and then they tell themselves they're weak. These people often beat themselves up for veering off course, but a lot of times it's not their fault at all - it's their physiology!

If they don't take time to improve this aspect, they'll likely follow the same pattern time and again. This can be the perfect set up for years of yo-yo diets. I seem to know a few things about yo-yo diets.

Tracking Macros

Beyond improving digestion, there are other things you can do to avoid obsessing over your new lifestyle. I personally was obsessed with dieting for too many years, and I never want to go back to that place.

If you want to have long term success on any plan, you have to learn how to make it your lifestyle instead of another diet you obsess over.

There are other keto leaders you may follow that tell you to not pay as much attention to macros in order to stop the diet obsession. I both agree and disagree strongly with this point of view.

So many keto hopefuls go into a keto plan with the desire of not tracking macros in order to avoid diet obsession. I completely understand that mindset since I'm the same girl who became so obsessive about tracking calories that once upon a time I actually had a screensaver on my work computer that told me how many calories I could eat during the entire month in order to hit my weight loss goal. I then subtracted each and every meal I ate from the monthly calorie total to see how many calories I had left in order to hit my monthly goal.

That right there - that's an entire new level of weight loss obsession!

To be fair, I also had a job where I didn't have much work to do, yet I had to always appear busy, so perhaps my diet obsession was something to fill the time.

Either way, that type of crazy obsession isn't sustainable for more than a few days, littlelone an entire month. Turns out, losing weight doesn't even come close to working that way.

While some people still say calories count on at least some level, counting calories isn't a plan that will work for most people long term. Also, there's absolutely no way an obsessive plan like I set up would ever work. Oh the things I could teach my twenty-something year old self.

I agree that you never want to get to this level of macro counting obsession. There is far more to do in life than worry this much about your diet. If you find yourself falling into this orthorexic pattern, "Stahp it Rahn!"

Stop now and take a deep breath before you find yourself being run over on the side of the road by your psychotic baby mama. If you agree to slowly back away from the calorie counting mindset, I'll agree to slowly back away from the bad *Jersey Shore* jokes.

With that being said, I do think you need at least a loose count on macros. This is especially important when you first begin a keto plan. How else do you know at which level of macros you'll succeed if you don't know where you start?

There are many who follow more of a lazy keto approach where they basically only count to 20 grams of carbs each day; then they eat protein and fat to feel good. This is a method that could work for you. If you're following this plan and you're getting the results you want, then stick with it. It's a great method to follow if it works for you. It's easy, and there isn't much to obsess over.

On the other hand, a lot of ketoers may not find long term success with this method.

While this may be the perfect approach to help them begin since going from the standard American diet of 300 plus carbs each day to only 20 carbs per day will be huge for a lot of people. Ultimately though, I believe a significant portion of ketoers will need to learn how to track macros at some point along the way.

Obviously it's important to track carbs. If you're only eating foods listed as low carb, it's pretty easy to blow out your carb allotment each day. Eating between 20 to 50 grams of carbs, depending on your personal carb tolerance for success, isn't a lot of carbs. If you're also eating some of the keto fun foods, like peanut butter or fat bombs, those foods can add up to 20 to 50 carbs very quickly.

This means if you're eating low carb foods that others suggest for a keto plan, you can see how not at least tracking carbs can get you into trouble pretty quickly. If at the same time you add too much fat to a plan where you eat too many carbs, that's the perfect recipe for weight gain.

You're probably not this far into this book looking for ways to gain weight. That's not the intention of most keto dieters.

To be quite frank, when I first began low carb, I was sick of tracking everything! In the past there were times I thought way too much about my diet. By the time I hit my highest weight in 2014, I was over it.

I was over diets, I was over restriction, and I was over my constant weight battle. While I was ready to throw in the towel on weight loss entirely, I needed to think about my health. I overcame my diet crazed ways and figured out how to find success without obsession.

I finally found success sans diet obsession by starting a handwritten food journal. Writing down what you eat leads to far greater success for most people. If you're not recording what you eat in some type of food journal, you need to start!

I kept my food journal simple by writing down the food I ate right after each meal. All I wrote next to the food was the amount of carbs in that meal. I never weighed my food to the exact gram, but I learned approximate serving sizes, so I was close enough. Once I hit my carb allotment for the day, I focussed on fat and protein friendly foods to help with satiation.

If that's all of the tracking you want to do, test to see if this method works for you. The key to success is staying consistent. Be sure you're writing down the food you eat right before or after you eat it. It's so easy to forget something you ate by the end of the day, and that could be a snack that could put you over your carb limit for the day.

If you're not seeing results only by tracking only carbs, then it might be time for you to pay more attention to fat and protein. It's really easy to track all of the macros you eat each day in an app like Cronometer.

I personally believe the next most important macro to pay attention to is fat. This is mostly because many people starting out on a keto diet, or even those well into their plan, aren't getting the results they want because they're not eating enough fat.

This is a controversial keto topic that varies from expert to expert. You'll hear many well respected experts tell you if you have fat to burn on your body, you shouldn't eat even an ounce of extra fat. Unfortunately this leaves many ketoers left hung out to dry after not getting results on their keto diet. They can't understand why they cut carbs, calories and fat so low, yet they're still not finding consistent results.

I'll give you a hint ... it's because they cut carbs, calories and fat so low.

I agree with cutting out carbs; that's pretty basic.

However, when most dieters who've restricted their bodies of nutrients for too long cut too far back on calories from fat, their bodies hold onto their stored fat. We haven't evolved much past the caveman days of famine or feast. Back then it was dangerous to let go of stored body fat without enough nutritional fat coming in.

If a keto expert, or even someone on the message boards named TracyandBrian, told you to eat low fat on a diet that by definition is high fat, but their advice didn't work for you, don't give up on keto entirely.

Come to the tasty side of keto where you're allowed to eat fat to satiation.

This doesn't mean you get to shovel unlimited amounts of fat down your throat. This is especially true if you still haven't improved how your body digests fat. But once you're ready to come over to this side of the diet, you get to eat enough fat to feel like an actual human.

I already know your next question: How much fat should I eat to find success?

Since this is all so individualized, I can't give you an exact number. While this macro will vary from person to person, if you add up your macros for the day and you're only coming up with 60 or 70 grams of fat for the entire day, you're not eating enough fat.

I sometimes eat this much fat in only one meal. I would feel completely malnourished if I only ate 60 or 70 total grams of fat over the course of most days.

My typical fat consumption each day is at least in the triple digits. Keep in mind, I took precautions necessary to help my body digest fat well, and I'm an active person. This means your number may not be quite as high.

This is something you'll have to test for yourself to see results. Don't be afraid to test triple digits just because there are so many experts telling you to eat a low fat keto diet.

Protein is actually the last macro I pay attention to and adjust if I'm not seeing results. Of course this is something else that will vary from person to person.

I've never been a big fan of protein rich meals, so I don't tend to overdo protein. This means I never really had to pay attention to protein until I got really close to my goal weight.

Once you're within ten pounds or so of your goal weight, it can be hard to get those last few pounds off. Sometimes you have to pay really close attention to what you're eating to bust through those last ten pounds. Keep in mind, even if you're not at those last ten pounds, some sensitive people can get kicked out of ketosis if they overdo protein at any point, so pay more attention to this macro and reel it in if you think this applies to you.

If you do decide to track carb, fat and protein macros, keep in mind that you don't have to be obsessive. Macro perfection is never the goal. You'll want to stay close to the numbers where you get results, but you still want to listen to your body and give it what it's asking for, even when it doesn't fit into the macros you set for yourself.

Maybe one day you need a few extra berries to feel good, while other days you might feel weak or shaky and decide you need more chicken to feel better. Listen to your body without veering too far off your plan. You have the macros there to help guide you, but never become a slave to those macros where you don't feel good day to day because you're being too restrictive.

Once you get into your keto groove with macros, this is when some people can stop tracking; at least for a little while. After some time following macros, you'll instinctively know what to eat to feel good.

The good thing here is you learned how to count macros, so at any time if you aren't getting the results you want, you can go back to tracking to see where you are, and what you need to tweak. Use macro counting as a tool to help figure out where you need to be for success, and use it again anytime your plan needs to be tweaked for the results you want.

More Stop Obsessing Tactics

So far we've reviewed a lot when it comes to obsessing less by improving digestion and counting macros. Believe it or not, I still have a few more suggestions that can help you ditch diet mentality forever, while easing into a keto lifestyle without obsession.

Let's start with this jewel of information I know many of you need to hear: **Quit jumping from plan to plan.**

Take time to learn how to make adjustments according to what you're monitoring, be it your physiology, blood ketones or even macros. You don't need a brand new plan; you really just need to learn how to work with your body instead of against it.

It's interesting to note this very sentiment is how my website, Eating Fat is the New Skinny, began.

I have a dear friend who I've known since the mid 2000's. She's been around to long enough see my struggles with weight loss first hand.

If you remember the story about my foray into diet pills, she's actually the same friend I ran into at the doctor's office because she was trying out the same prescription diet pills as me. She has also had a bit of a struggle with her weight over the years I've known her.

Since she's been around to witness my ultimate low carb transformation, she texts quite often to help her figure out strategies that will help her lose weight. She's what some people refer to as an askhole.

No, I didn't misspell that word, nor would I call my dear friend a derogatory name like that. I did call her an askhole - with a K.

This is because she's been messaging me for years asking for the same advice over and over. I spent a lot of time texting her back the right information, assuming she would take the slow and steady approach I offered.

Every few months I'd hear back from her again about how she's gained even more weight, and she wanted to know how to start. Again.

Since we've had many other texting conversations in between, it wasn't like I could just say "see previous texts." I'd text her again from scratch with all of this great information that in the back of my mind I knew she wouldn't follow. Again.

I'll admit, I eventually became frustrated with her askhole ways, and may or may not have been a little snappy over texts. I try to keep my composure, especially with friends, but her health was deteriorating right before my eyes. I hoped a dose of tough love might do the trick.

It was from this frustration that I started blogging the steps I took so I could help others that didn't know where to start. I needed somewhere to house my blogs, so that's when I started my website, and those blogs eventually turned into a book, a la Carrie's articles in *Sex and the City*. Her's just might be a tad more popular than my book though, you know, since Candace Bushnell had that show on HBO, plus a few movies.

I wonder if HBO wants to follow the life of a yo-yo dieter? Is it embarrassing to admit that I'd watch that show?

If you have the HBO hook up, I'd love to be played by Jessica Simpson since everything that girl touches turns to gold. She's also struggled with her weight just like me, so it's believable.

Back to the suggestion at hand - quit chasing the shiny new diet in the room and follow through on your commitment. If you don't see results after that first or second week, that doesn't mean you should uproot your efforts and abandon ship for something new. You need to have patience and allow the plan you chose time to work.

Of course this doesn't mean if you're showing signs of poor fat digestion that you should push through and keto on because that's the plan you chose. Be smart about this.

If you're not showing signs of poor fat digestion, you need to quit looking to the scale for results, and then giving up after only one or two weeks, or even one or two months, because the weight isn't falling off like you expected. This all takes patience and time. If you're not seeing results, then you need to keep digging into what might be holding you back instead of giving up and chasing a brand new plan that someone else swears by.

Keep in mind, your body may need time to adjust, and that could be why you're not seeing the results you want on the scale.

Your body also could be adjusting with improved bone density or more muscle. If this is the case, you might not see the number on the scale go down. This is especially true if intermittent fasting is part of your plan.

While most people celebrate the scale moving down with a happy dance, it's important to note that gaining muscle or bone density is huge! Let's all do a happy dance for a better body composition since that's really what you want anyway.

You may not understand that's what you want since you've been trained to only look for results on the scale, but trust me, those are the results you want.

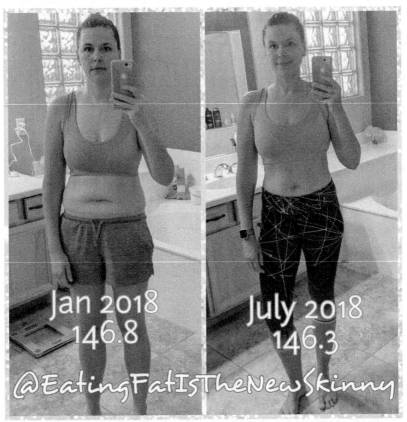

Jan 2018
146.8

July 2018
146.3

@EatingFatIsTheNewSkinny

Same scale weight, but down 2 sizes thanks to body recompositioning!

Better body composition makes your clothes fit better, and gives you a healthier body. The scale moving down each week doesn't necessarily mean fat loss; it only means weight loss. Is that loss on the scale water weight, muscle, bone density or actual fat?

The problem is, most people don't know what type of scale loss they're celebrating.

You need to use other factors to determine if your plan is working. Just because the scale didn't jump down as you expected one week, you can't throw in the towel and say keto doesn't work. There are so many other factors to consider. Constantly chasing the newest and shiniest diet out there will never provide the results you want. This pattern will only lead you to more frustration, more yo-yo diets and more long term health problems.

Now is a good time to instill in yourself that results will take time; most likely a lot of time and patience is key.

Also, keep in mind that results are rarely linear. You may have a big loss one week, and then gain a pound the next.

This is another reason relying on only the scale for results is bad news bears. I know many of you are still sticking your fingers in your ears when I tell you that. If you insist on using the scale for results each week, at the very least you have to have patience and understand that number won't necessarily go down each and every week just because you're following a keto plan. Deal?

And PS, I'm back to answering my friend's texts frustration free because she finally took my advice seriously. She even joined one of my Keto Challenges! Below is a snippet of how her time went during the 21 day challenge. As you read this, keep in mind these are the changes she experienced by following keto the right way for only three weeks! In three weeks, she completely changed her health trajectory and had all of these amazing wins!

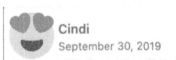

Cindi
September 30, 2019

First I want thank Nissa Batson-Graun for never giving up on me, she has been wanting me to try keto for years. I think for me was fear of letting go of the sugar. I am addicted to sugar and like anyone who has an addiction to drugs, alchohol etc, there is a fear of letting it go. I know if I don't let go of the sugar, Sugar will kill me. I have a beautiful 7 year old son that I have to be here for and a wonderful hubby to. I lost me parents as a child and if it's within my power I will not do that to him. Doing this challenge I have completely given up Tea with milk and a lot of sugar and if you know me you know that would never happen. So I am completely caffine free. I have given up rice, potatoes, bread, (we are Puerto Rican that is almost our complete diet lol) pasta, and candy. I feel great! Before the challenge I felt swollen, my knee's hurt, my joints hurt even my elbows hurt. Now I don't feel swollen and I could even wear my wedding ring again comfortably. We all have heard and read Nissa say it's not so much the number on the scale it's how you feel and how your clothes fit, well I had a pair of jeans that I had that I bought that didn't fit when I bought them, but almost fit, then I kept gaining weight and the jeans were barely fitting. Well we live in Illinois and it has been a little cooler these last few days so I found these jeans in the closet and I was like what the heck let me try them on, they not only fit but I could zipper them and button them! 😺 🎤 Wow I was so happy! So I am down 14.3 lbs with the challenge and even though I didn't win the prize, my prize is

Quit Expecting A Set Loss Each Week

That brings me to another important point about how not to obsess on your new keto plan. ***Quit expecting to lose a set amount of weight each week.***

I literally just told you that your results on the scale will not be linear. Did you forget already?

While setting goals is a great approach, becoming upset with yourself because you didn't hit the two pound weight loss goal you set for yourself this week is silly. If you did everything you could to hit the two pound goal, but it didn't happen, you need to learn how to be kind to yourself. Never beat yourself up because you didn't hit a goal you had set for yourself.

Instead of relying so much on the scale to prove what you're doing is working, focus more on how you feel.

Do you love the way you're eating? Do you have tons of energy? Are your clothes fitting better? Have you taken progress pictures so you can compare them to the pictures you'll take again next month?

These are the things that really matter. Not hitting a specific amount of weight lost each week really isn't all that important in the grand scheme of things. Adding up small wins, like feeling great or noticing looser fitting clothing, are the things that matter long term.

Perhaps instead of relying on a weekly scale weight, you need to measure your results more on a monthly basis. If you become obsessive or upset if the results don't go how you wanted on a weekly basis, then measuring on a weekly basis is a good way to derail your results.

The same thing is true for measurements.

Measurements are a great way to know if you're losing body fat, but you won't see changes every week. Again, this is where patience comes in, so focusing more on how you feel and making sure you're sticking to your plan in order to see those month to month results is what's important. It's definitely way more important than the number shown on the scale each week.

If you can't seem to get past your undying need for stepping on the scale, you can try weight averaging in order to see a month to month trend. This can be a great method to see how your body is losing weight. With weight averaging, you're no longer only relying on one inaccurate number to measure your progress that week. You'll have more data to see how your weight loss efforts are trending over time.

You still need to pay attention to your mindset. It might actually be even a little more important to pay attention to your mindset before you try weight averaging.

With weight averaging, you'll weigh yourself once each day. If that's too often for you, you can even try a pattern like 3 or 4 days each week. Just be consistent.

Since you have to weigh yourself more often, if seeing a number you don't want to see mentally drains you or causes self cruelty, don't use this method! If you can't patiently wait a few weeks to determine your real results, this is not a method for you.

Of course, true fat loss takes patience in general. Since you need to learn to be patient anyway, this method can be great to consider since you'll see more information than just a weekly number that will fluctuate from week to week.

The way weight averaging works is you weigh yourself everyday and record the number. At the end of the week, you add up all of the weights and divide by 7. That will be your average weight for that week.

You'll do the same thing the next week and beyond.

If you only choose to weigh in 4 days each week, then you'll only divide the total week's weight by 4. Then compare your average weight each week instead of just relying on weighing in once each week, and going by that number.

One reason this is a better method is you're getting more of the story than just one day's worth of data. If you weigh in at 150 pounds after your first week of keto, and then weigh in at 151 pounds after your second week, this would cause a lot of people to feel hopeless because they tried so hard only to gain a pound.

Sometimes when you average numbers throughout the week, your weight average for week 1 may have actually been 150 pounds. Your weight at the end of week two could still be 151 pounds, but maybe you're showing an average for the week of only 149 lbs.

This means while you went up one pound on the scale from week one to week two, your average is down a pound. The pound you went up when only checking in one day each week could have been extra water your body was holding onto, or maybe you just have to poop.

Looking at the average from week to week will provide more accuracy than just weighing in once each week and using that as the only number you use to determine if your plan is working.

When you look at weight averages, some days your weight may be higher, and some days it may be lower than the previous week. As long as that week to week average is trending down most weeks, you know you're doing the right things to move the scale in the right direction.

I also feel like with this method you can really learn to use the scale weight as data. Quit weighing in once each week and feeling either absolutely ecstatic, or all doom and gloom based on a number that could be artificially inflated. Maybe you consumed just a few too many carbs the night before, and your body is holding onto a little extra water weight.

That water weight could very well be gone in an hour or two. In fact, did you know your weight can fluctuate at least in a five pound range each day? What you weigh at 7 am could be one to five pounds more or less than what you weigh at 4 pm on the same day.

Do you think you gained or lost five pounds of fat between 7am and 4pm? Nope! Fat loss will never work that way.

Remember - this method is supposed to help you learn patience, and help you see the bigger picture. If it's only leading to more weight loss obsession, step away from the scale!

Not even knowing good data about your body is worth the kind of mental anguish the scale can bring if you don't understand how to use the daily numbers as data instead of ways to punish yourself for not ketoing hard enough.

Learn How To Cook

Another way to not obsess about your new keto lifestyle is to learn how to cook so the food you're eating actually tastes good. I already touched on this earlier in this chapter, so I won't talk too much about it here; but this one is important.

When I tried low carb in the past, I spent so much time thinking about what to eat next because I wasn't giving my body the nutrients it needs when I was simply pulling through the drive thru, ordering two low quality burgers, and removing the buns.

Sure that's low carb, and sure you can still see results with this dirty keto lifestyle, but how will you feel? And how long will your results last with low quality food that doesn't contain a lot of nutrients?

If you're seriously considering these questions, "Stahp it Rahn!" I can assure you that you won't feel great, and your results, as well as your low carb plan, won't last long. I have plenty of experience to back up this claim.

When you feel hunger on a low carb diet, your body might be searching for more nutrients, not necessarily more food. If you're only eating low quality food most of the time because you never learned how to cook higher quality food, then you'll likely be hungry most of the time, and you'll always obsess over your next meal.

I know this can be hard for some people. We all lead busy lives. Not only does cooking take time, but then there's all of the dishes and prep work you also need to make time for. Trust me, I felt the same way, especially after I became a mother and taking care of a newborn consumed my life.

I put some thought into it, and realized the time it took for me to pack up the baby, drive to a drive thru, order food and drive home was about the same amount of time it would have taken to stay home and cook a meal I would enjoy much more since my homemade meals use higher quality ingredients.

If you're accustomed to low quality food, trust me when I say this - when you start providing your body high quality, nutrient dense food that it can break down properly, you'll start preferring the food you can cook at home as well.

As a reformed fast food junkie, I never thought this would become a truth for me. I learned how to cook delicious keto meals, and turns out, I now understand why people long for home cooked meals over fast food junk.

If you're still in the mindset that cooking at home is too much work, and you don't have time, definitely check out the Keto Decoded Cooking Course I mentioned earlier. Not only do we have plenty of recipes and cooking demonstrations to help you learn how to make delicious keto meals, but there's an entire educational section in the course where you'll learn easy hacks to make keto cooking much easier. Many of these hacks will also save you time. Since time is money, you're actually saving money by taking the course.

If you're not quite ready for keto, or if you prefer a low carb lifestyle, we have a low carb Cooking Decoded Course set up as well.

Learn Even More

The last tip I have to not obsess over your new keto lifestyle is to stay educated. You're taking a great first step by reading books like this, but you need to stay on top of new information regarding health and diet.

Most people who obsess over their plans are usually the same people that are desperate to see results, but they're likely not getting results because they're following along with what everyone else is doing instead taking the time to learn how to work with their own body to see results.

People who become informed about their bodies and their situations don't need to obsess over a plan that's not working for them. If something doesn't go as planned, they know the next step to take to get back on track because they've taken the time to research and become informed.

If you're just throwing caution to the wind and jumping on the keto bandwagon because so many others are getting results, but you haven't taken time to do your own research, that sounds like a plan for diet disaster.

Beyond this book, I have an entire list of resources at the end of the book for you to get started with furthering your keto education. Of course, you can check out my other books or even our podcast. My co-host, T.C. Hale, also has a phenomenal book on Amazon called *Kick Your Fat in the Nuts*. If you haven't read that one yet, your health education has yet to begin!

It's so important not to obsess over your plan in order to escape diet mentality. If you do become obsessive, take a step back and tell yourself no! Smack your hand if that's what it takes. I sometimes have to tap my dog's nose when I tell her no, so maybe try that.
While she's pretty stubborn, she responds to even a light tap. Do whatever it takes to not fall into the diet obsession trap.

Chapter 5: My Big Fat Saga

If you're following a keto plan and hoping to find lasting success, eating more fat is vital.

I've already stated my controversial view several times throughout this book that *a lot of ketoers need to eat more fat* if they run into a weight loss stall, not less.

Even if you have fat to burn on your body, that stored fat won't be easy to access if you're not taking in enough nutritional fat to even get into ketosis in the first place.

Sorry other keto experts; it's just a fact of keto life.

I'm actually not sure why so many experts insist if you have fat to burn on your body, that you shouldn't take in additional nutritional fat. Sure, *you don't want to chug fat like there's no tomorrow …* but nobody's telling you to do that.

Perhaps these other experts only want to clue you into the very basics when it comes to a keto plan. I'm using this book to help you dig deeper into reasons why eating more fat on a keto diet may not be working for you now. I don't want to leave you high and dry, so I'll even share a few embarrassing stories to help you learn how to improve any issues you may have while following a proper high fat keto plan.

My Big Fat Life

Let me welcome you to the saga that was my life when I took steps to improve the way my body digested fat. And yes, I just called it a saga, because if you read the blog I wrote a few years ago titled *About that Noxema Girl,* you know I had to take what some might consider drastic steps to improve the way my body digested fat before I could move from low carb into a keto plan.

You've already read a lot about digestion throughout this book. In case you haven't realized it yet, digesting the food you eat is important! If your body is storing the food you eat as toxins instead of digesting that food and using it for energy as it should, hopefully you can see how that will become a huge problem for not only weight loss, but also for health.

While I talk a lot about digestion, as well as the steps I took to improve digestion, sometimes that all won't mean very much to you without learning how to put all of this talk into action.

Sometimes hearing someone else's story can help you figure out if what we're talking about is something you need to consider for yourself, and learning the steps I used might help guide you on the path to improving fat digestion for yourself.

Before I found the book *Kick Your Fat in the Nuts,* I never really understood what digestion meant. I mean, you eat, you poop and you eat again, right? Or in my case, where I was unknowingly severely constipated, I ate, I ate, I ate and on the 7th day I pooped; or at least some similar pattern.

Sure, I saw the Activia commercials with Jamie Lee Curtis, but those were geared toward my grandparents, so I never put a second thought into digestion; at least until I came across the book and learned there is so much more that goes into digestion.

After seeing myself throughout the entire book, I realized my digestion could use a little work. The book finally explained some of the lifelong ailments I experienced and my weight and health struggles all began to make a little more sense.

Signs of Poor Fat Digestion

Some of the clues I learned that meant I had poor fat digestion include the cystic acne I had since I was a teenager, as well as the nausea and intense cravings for carbs every time I began a low carb plan.

I also had bouts of painful gas, my stool was light in color and I had itchy skin, which became almost unbearable during pregnancy. There were some nights during pregnancy where I'd lay in bed and spend upwards of an hour itching my legs in a mad furor instead of getting a good night's rest.

Many of these symptoms I thought were a normal part of life; especially the carb cravings while on a low carb diet, and the painful gas I endured since I was a teenager. Well, at least the cravings part, because the really painful gas definitely wasn't normal.

There were times I'd be struck with so much pain in my lower abdomen that my entire life had to stop so I could hunch over in agony. While I was pretty sure that wasn't normal, the only way I knew how to escape the pain was to chew a few Gas-X tablets for eventual relief, but those tablets never prevented future painful attacks. There were times the pain was so intense that I considered an ER visit.

Whenever I became nauseous on a low carb diet, I felt the need to immediately eat crackers or bread to feel better. I honestly believed this was something everyone experienced, or at least most women, since my husband never seemed to deal with this issue.

I chalked it up to men being more primal and thriving off meat, while women biologically needed more carbs. I'm not even sure how I came up with this hypothesis since I don't recall reading it in any of the diet books I devoured; but I was sure I was correct in my hypothesis.

In the past, it was difficult to make it more than four or five days on a low carb plan without the terrible nausea where I had to break my plan to eat crackers. Needless to say, the strong urge to eat carbs killed any progress I made.

There were times I pushed through longer than the first week. In fact, one time I white knuckled my way through a 45 pound weight loss, but that was hard. Like, really really hard.

I pushed through because I wanted to look good in a bathing suit on a trip, but I didn't feel great most of the time. I also put the weight back on very rapidly once on the trip, and off the low carb plan. I packed two different sized shorts for that trip, and I barely squeezed into the larger size by the end.

I also often lacked energy on a low carb plan because my body wasn't breaking down the fat I ate as fuel. Since carbs were the only thing my body really understood how to utilize as fuel, eating more fat wasn't the answer. Still, everyone advised me to eat less carbs and more fat, so I kept trying to force a plan that wasn't right for my body.

Regarding persistent acne, I thought I was unlucky. As teenagers, we're told it's a normal part of life, and hormones and chocolate get the blame.

I dealt with non stop acne for years with over the counter solutions. When I still had this problem in my 20's, I called in the professionals and visited the dermatologist regularly, but my problem seemed to worsen over time.

The creams prescribed by dermatologists dried out my skin everywhere except the spots acne sprouted. My face was a war zone. I had spots of extremely dry skin, combined with large pus filled acne on my cheeks, around my mouth, on my forehead and sometimes right between my eyes; you know, the place everyone looks when you have a conversation.

It. Was. The. Worst.

I spent so many nights testing out different masks and other potions that were guaranteed to work, but in the end, only did more damage to my delicate skin.

I gave Accutane a whirl - more than once. If you haven't heard the story on Accutane, that's some scary stuff. Doctors who prescribe this medication make you agree to go on birth control. If you become pregnant while on Accutane, your baby would likely come out severely deformed. There's even a warning label with a pregnant lady on each pill with a bold red circle with a line through it. Pregnant women aren't even supposed to touch the package.

Since I had no current pregnancy plans, I thought what's the harm? I signed on the dotted line and took the prescription. Twice.

While my acne did clear up, this solution came along with severely dry skin, especially around my mouth and nose. I resembled a clown when I applied makeup because of all of the peeling skin.

My eyes were so dry that I wouldn't have been able to cry even if my dog died. The inside of my nose was so dry that my boogers felt like ice picks stabbing the inside of my nose. These symptoms went on for months.

Since this was the solution to ending cystic acne forever, I dealt with the side effects.

Accutane did clear up my acne … for about a year. After a few more years of dealing with rebound cystic acne, I was back on this prescription that I was previously told was my forever solution. When I think of forever, I think of much longer than a year. The makers of Accutane have a much different version of forever than I do.

If you've never dealt with acne like this, you have no idea the effects of cysts all over your face can have your self esteem. I was so desperate to get rid of these awful, pussy bumps all over my face that I went on a medication … twice … that did horrid things to my body.

In the back of my mind, I was terrified I was doing bad things to my reproductive system with this medication. While I had no plans for babies at the time, I knew I wanted to be a mother someday. It's sad that I potentially risked healthy pregnancies just to get something most people take for granted - clear skin.

Thankfully I went on to have two healthy kids. While I don't know if Accutane affects future fertility, I always feared it could have at the time I took this drug.

These are some of the symptoms I dealt with due to poor fat digestion. Let's also review some life events that led to poor fat digestion since these are pretty common among many yo-yo dieters. You may even see yourself in at least some of these scenarios.

How Poor Fat Digestion Can Happen

Thankfully I never really ate a low fat diet since I figured out early on while attempting a low fat plan that I didn't feel great. While I typically ate foods that were a little higher in fat than the 80's allowed, I wasn't eating the right kinds of fat.

Of course, I shouldn't blame myself for this since as dieters we can never get a straight answer as to which kind of fat is the healthy kind of fat. One expert says monounsaturated, while another expert says polyunsaturated.

Thankfully none of the experts pinpoint trans fat as healthy; but since I considered myself a junk food junkie, I was eating plenty of trans fats. Back then, and even now, a lot of experts will tell you to steer clear of saturated fats too.

So many experts; so much bad information!

Another reason I dealt with poor fat digestion is I spent so many years in the low calorie dieting world. I was constantly on and off programs like Weight Watchers, Jenny Craig and SlimFast. These programs are designed to cut calories very low in order to find weight loss success. While perhaps these programs don't claim to be low fat by design, if you're cutting calories as low as suggested, you'll be eating plenty of low fat foods since fat is such a calorically dense food.

There are 9 calories in each gram of fat, compared to only 4 calories in each gram of carbohydrate or protein. If you're on a plan designed to cut calories, you're on a plan that's going to cut fat - even if it's a low calorie, low carb or keto plan.

When I followed all of these low calorie plans, I ate all of the recommended 'healthy' whole grains. Guess which food does a great job at sludging up bile - yep, healthy whole grains.

When bile gets sludgy, your body starts storing the fat you eat as toxins, and those toxins get shoved into your fat cells. Basically, you could get fat no matter how low calories go.

Along with the 'healthy' whole grains, I could never quite kick my addiction to fried potato love, like chips or french fries. Even if I was following a low calorie plan, I found ways to incorporate these foods daily. I simply made sure they fit into my daily calories.

These are the types of fat I was eating that aren't ideal for better fat digestion. This doesn't even mention that high carb foods that are also high fat foods are public enemy #1 when it comes to weight gain. Just think about all of the foods that make most people gain weight quickly:

Big Macs and fried chicken and French fries, oh my!

All foods that are both high in fat, while also being high in carbs.

When I was in between diets, since at some point I became an insane lunatic on any diet when I could no longer take the restriction, I've been known to eat an entire bag of potato chips, and I don't mean the single serving bag.

I've definitely eaten a family size bag of chips more than once while in between diets. If you've been a yo-yo dieter at any point in your life, I know you can relate to long periods of restriction, followed by at least short periods of junk food binges.

Someone recently asked me if I was ever a binge eater and my natural response was no. Looking back, I'm not sure why I immediately replied no since eating an entire bag of chips in one sitting is definitely a good binge. I never purged, so maybe that's the reason I was so quick to say no.

I've always lumped binging and purging together. Thinking back through my yo-yo history, I've been a binger since at least age 12. I remember walking to our local Walgreens with my step sisters, where we'd each buy our own large bags of Doritos. Each of us would eat the entire bag in one sitting. I was definitely a binger from early on, and once again, I never even realized that about myself.

Needless to say, eating this way caused a few chronic health conditions. At the time, I never associated the way I felt with the food I ate, but now I understand the connection. Some of the health problems that resulted from my poor diet I tried to improve for decades with over the counter medications.

Just as the food I ate contributed to sludgy bile, these medications, both over the counter and prescription, were also doing their part to sludge up my bile flow. Masking the health symptoms I had with medications may have helped me in the moment, but over the long term, they made the problem worse.

When I read *Kick Your Fat in the Nuts* and began the steps to improve digestion, I figured out I also had some of the chemistry imbalances listed in the book. I didn't understand how improving these would help me lose weight, but I was desperate since none of my old calorie cutting tricks were doing the trick.

I gave these new methods the old college try. I was pretty much a brown noser in college, so my college try may have been a little bit more involved than most.

My personal chemistry imbalances included:

- A Catabolic imbalance
- Low blood pressure
- Saliva and urine pH's not in appropriate ranges
- The fat digestion issues I listed above

Before moving onto a keto diet, I was low carb for the first year. This was mostly because I had no idea keto even existed. Believe me, if back then I knew about a diet that could supercharge my results, I would've tried that diet the very next day.

I'm thankful I didn't know about keto at the time because with poor digestion, combined with imbalances like a catabolic imbalance and low blood pressure, I would have failed keto miserably. I'd likely still be stuck in the world of yo-yo diets to this day.

Keto can exacerbate these imbalances. My body needed those extra carbs allowed on a low carb plan in order to find success that first year. Not only did I feel good while finding success, but I actually found a lot of success that first year. I was able to eat a considerable amount of carbs to go along with that success.

I lost somewhere around 70 pounds the first year by lowering carbs to a low carb level, combined with taking steps to improve digestion and balance body chemistry. If you're in the same place as far as digestion or imbalances are concerned, don't be afraid to take a step back and do what you need to do to feel good when starting this lifestyle.

A strict ketogenic diet isn't the only way to have success. You should never force a plan where you don't feel good. That's really the theme of this book - finding the right plan for you while also feeling like a normal human being who's not obsessed with a diet plan.

We talk about how to tell which plan is right for you in our Keto Decoded Courses. If you decide you're not quite ready for keto, we show you how to find success with a low carb plan. Of course, I'll continue to walk you through some of these steps throughout the remainder of this book as well.

How I Improved Fat Digestion

When I followed a low carb plan the first year, I began improving sludgy bile by adding Beet Flow with meals. After a few days of adding this supplement, I tried a Beet Flow Flush.

Holy nausea Batman!

I felt like I had to lie down in the fetal position. All of the toxins that were previously stored in fat cells were getting stirred up and causing incredible nausea.

Ever the dieter on a mission, I stuck with the flush through the nausea. I did a few more flushes after that for good measure. Well, also for better bile flow.

Over time, Beet Flow helped with nausea, so I was able to stay on track to improve fat digestion long term. I also added coconut yummies after meals to help my body become accustomed to more fats in my diet.

My body was deprived of healthy fats for so long that even though I wasn't following keto at the time, I needed to add extra fat in order to help my body recognize that sufficient fat was coming in. This sent a signal to my body that it was OK to let go of stored body fat.

In case you're unsure which kind of fat to focus on if you have sludgy bile, coconut oil is one of the best fats you can add to meals.

Coconut oil doesn't require strong bile flow to break it down, which means it will be easier for you to digest. When you add coconut oil to a meal when digestion is already happening, it will be even easier for you to break down. If you are experiencing poor fat digestion, but you need to add more fat to your diet so your body will let go of stored fat, coconut oil is a great choice.

When I began low carb, I used almost pure coconut oil with the coconut yummy recipe. They're a little strange at first, but coconut yummies are something you'll learn to like if you eat them enough.

If you can't get down with almost pure coconut oil, maybe try some of the recipes on my website that are heavy in coconut oil, like minty melts or orange chocolate fat bombs. Those varieties have chocolate and extracts to make them more palatable. Actually, I love both of these fat bombs, so stating that they're only palatable is doing these recipes a disservice.

Since I was low carb for almost a full year prior to stumbling upon keto, I was able to ramp up fat intake over time instead of rushing the process like a lot of ketoers do. I think this, along with the ability to still eat some carbs with meals, helped cement a low carb lifestyle for me.

In previous dieting attempts, I'd always planned to go back to eating something close to the diet I had before I began my new plan. Allowing myself time to improve digestion, while slowly changing out the foods I ate, helped me learn to love this new way of eating to the point where I no longer wanted the junk food I lived on for so long.

I'm not saying that you too should follow low carb for a year before you move onto keto. We're all different and we all have different needs. If you're struggling with fat digestion, it's time to go back to low carb for at least a little while. Take time to ramp up your fat intake over time, while simultaneously taking steps to improve how your body digests fat. This can help you succeed with keto long term when you decide to give it a go; if you make that decision at all. There's no shame in sticking with a low carb plan if you decide that's a lifestyle you enjoy.

Improving Fat Digestion Improved Chronic Health Issues

As I took this year to improve digestion with supplements and food choices, I noticed many chronic health problems I dealt with for decades were improving. I no longer experienced frequent migraines, and even my dull headaches were less frequent and not as painful as they once were.

The diabetic blood sugar levels I had after pregnancy lowered to a normal range after only a few months of following this plan.

That's pretty much unheard of in the medical world where they rely on medications and a diet filled with 'healthy' whole grains and fruit to help lower blood sugar.

I also noticed the anxiety, painful gas and occasional depression I dealt with for decades were just gone.

The one ailment that was not improving quite as much as I'd hoped was my acne. While it did clear up somewhat, I still had more breakouts than I would have preferred.

Obviously I preferred no breakouts, but acne was such a huge part of my existence for so long, that I didn't think getting rid of my scarlet letter for good was even feasible. I truly thought embarrassing acne would be something I'd have to deal with for life.

Still, I wanted to improve my complexion as much as I could. I did more research and re-read the parts of *Kick Your Fat in the Nuts* that dealt with un-sludging sludgy bile.

While I was still following the routine of Beet Flow with meals and occasional Beet Flow Flushes, the book and support group also recommended a supplement called Xeneplex. While I steadily lost weight with diet changes and digestive supplements, I decided Xeneplex was the next right step for me to improve acne.

I was ready to give Xeneplex a try! Then I saw the price. Xeneplex, the possible cure to my acne woes, was $89 for only 10 pills.

Yikes. I was already spending more money than I was comfortable with on supplements with my regimen of Beet flow, HCL, digestive enzymes and Bio C. It was difficult to justify adding another $89 in supplements, even if it was only a one time purchase.

I was also skeptical after the Accutane experience. That was supposed to be my cystic acne savior for life, and after two rounds it seemed my acne had only gotten worse. I had trouble buying into the hype of anything that claimed it would help me, be it prescribed or natural.

Then I thought about all of the money I still spent on creams, fancy face washes, and other solutions that were supposed to help that obviously weren't really helping. I realized if this really was the solution that was going to help long term, it was completely worth $89, so I ordered that little red box with only 10 pills.

My next hesitation with Xeneplex came with the supplement instructions. I guess I never really paid attention to what Xeneplex actually was. If you're not sure what it is at this point either, it's a suppository. If that still means nothing to you, that means you have to stick it in your butt. And not only do you have to pull out the vaseline, lube up your finger and shove a pill in your butt, but you also had to hold it there for as long as you could muster.

While I thought all of my anxiety cleared up long ago, I definitely had at least a little anxiety about using butt pills. Sure, I was cut in half a year prior since my baby was delivered by C-section, but for some reason that seemed insignificant compared to popping a pill into an area designated as exit only.

I got over my fears and took the long, lonely walk to the bathroom to give this Xeneplex thing a go. Turns out, it wasn't so bad.

Sure, it's not a process I'd prefer an audience for, and maybe I can only talk about it now because I'm hiding behind the pages of this book, but this routine came with good news. I followed this process a few times, and then followed each time up with a Beet Flow Flush the next day. After not too long of following these instructions, my acne disappeared!

This self esteem crushing problem I dealt with for so long was finally gone. I was still at least a little skeptical due to the Accutane experience, but I'm happy to report my long and lonely walk to the bathroom was five years ago. My acne problem was resolved, and never returned. I don't even deal with pimples around that special time of the month like many women do.

I never even dreamed my skin could be so clear. For so long I was the girl who would never leave the house without a full face of makeup because I was so desperate to cover up acne.

These days I barely wear makeup. I hardly even wash my face. I know that's not a great habit, but I only mention it because back in the days cystic acne ruled my face, there were days I washed my face up to three times per day in an attempt to find relief.

Now there are days I go without washing it at all. Improving fat digestion is truly the miracle I sought out for decades. I realize as a health professional I'm not supposed to call these things a miracle, but cystic acne no longer crushing my self esteem and ruling my life is a miracle in my book.

I go into this in a lot more detail in the *About that Noxema Girl* blog, so if you haven't read it yet, now's your chance. I guarantee you'll learn a few things, but more importantly, you'll laugh. Yes, you'll be laughing at my expense, but I'm OK with it because I no longer deal with cystic acne, *and* I'm back to the days where that special area I referenced earlier is back to exit only.

About Those Supplements

When people first hear about the digestive supplements I reference throughout this book, one of the first questions asked is how long do I need to take the supplements?

Of course most people don't want to take supplements in the first place, so once they decide the supplements might help them, they want a timeline. Believe me, I was fully on board with that thought process as well.

The truth is, I can't tell you how long you'll take the supplements, or even which combo of supplements you'll need because we're all different and each of our bodies are screwed up a little differently.

As you may have guessed from this book, mine was pretty screwed up. Twenty plus years as a yo-yo dieter tends to mess a person up like that.

While I can't tell you how long you'll require supplements, I can tell you that I ended up taking the digestive supplements Beet Flow and HCL for around a year. I also only required one box of Xeneplex to help improve extra sludgy bile.

There were times over that year that I tested removing all of the supplements from my routine, but it didn't take long for some of my undesirable symptoms to return. That's how I knew I needed to keep them around a little longer.

Right around that year mark, I became pregnant with my second child. Since doctors scare pregnant women away from taking almost anything in pill form, I decided against taking any of the supplements during pregnancy. While I was pregnant, baby #2 brought along severe heartburn, so I backslid as far as digestion was concerned. I started the supplement routine again as soon as I recovered from birth.

There you have my full story about impaired fat digestion, and the process I took to get sludgy bile moving again. Hopefully this fat digestion saga helps you better understand some of the steps you may need to take to improve sludgy bile.

When I began, there was some confusion that came along with this process, but I learned as I went along. I gave you some starting points in this chapter, and referenced some great reading materials, so you can start there.

Of course, if you're following all of this information and you're still stuck, pop into the Eating Fat is the New Skinny Support Group with any questions you have. Remember, we all need to start our learning somewhere, so no question is a dumb question. If you have questions, others have the same questions. Please ask your questions so everyone can learn together.

C'mon, I just told an entire story about butt pills. Surely any questions you might have are at least a little less embarrassing.

Before I end this chapter, the real take home message is there is no such thing as magic weight loss pills. The supplements I reference are not magic, and randomly popping the supplements I used won't help you lose weight.

If you're strategic about this, and you use the right supplements for your body, the supplements do help improve digestion, which can be the magic you need. If your body no longer views the fat you eat as toxic, it will see the value of nutritional fat you have coming in, so it can release stored fat from your body.

Chapter 6: A Tale of Low Blood Pressure

How many of the *experts* you sought advice from on the keto message boards asked you about your blood pressure when you complained of headaches, dizziness, nausea or anxiety?

Likely not a single one.

I bet most of these *experts* shouted things like, "keto flu!" or "electrolytes!"

I know sarcasm is hard to pick up in a book, even when I use italics, so let me point out I don't think a lot of those people answering questions on the message boards are really keto experts. While many of these people mean well, most of those hanging out on the message boards are only everyday people who tried keto, and it helped them lose a few pounds. Many believe if something worked for them, then the exact steps they took must work for everyone else on the planet.

While this is far from the truth, and experts they are not, they are onto something. When you experience symptoms like headaches, dizziness, nausea or anxiety when you start keto, these symptoms could be attributed to what some refer to as the dreaded keto flu, which can be caused by low electrolytes.

What many of the message board experts don't understand is beginning a keto plan often results in peeing out many of the electrolytes your body holds onto when you're eating a higher amount of carbs. Once you drop carbs to ketogenic levels, you pee out electrolytes in large quantities, and this may cause your blood pressure to drop.

If you start a keto diet, and your blood pressure is already low from years of yo-yo diets, or perhaps you're not breaking down the food you eat well, you're pretty much screwed. Attempting a keto diet with low blood pressure can be downright disastrous!

Then again, even just going through life with low blood pressure can be disastrous.

While everyone in the mainstream warns of the dangers of high blood pressure, most stay mum when it comes to walking through life with low blood pressure. In fact, if you commonly have low blood pressure - quit walking through life. Take a break because I don't want you to pass out!

Just kidding; well, kind of. You could feel light headed when you have low blood pressure, so if that's you, be sure you're sitting down while reading this book.

Since not very many in the keto world discuss low blood pressure, and I happen to know a thing or two about low blood pressure, now is a good time for you to learn more. Just as with the last chapter, where I discussed poor fat digestion, for a good chunk of my life I also dealt with low blood pressure and all of the symptoms that come along with this issue no one discusses.

Before coming across this valuable information in *Kick Your Fat in the Nuts*, I never realized low blood pressure was a thing. I definitely never knew it was a problem that was wreaking havoc on all of my dieting attempts.

I also didn't understand low blood pressure was causing some of the health problems I began experiencing around the time I started my time in the low fat, low calorie dieting world as a preteen.

I do want to throw in a quick tangent here to note that while 12 years old is far too young to become part of this low calorie dieting world, I fear this is becoming the norm for kids who are even younger than this these days. This is a time when kids need adequate nutrition, particularly healthy fats for a healthy brain, not more restriction.

As this healthy fat message makes its way to the mainstream more and more, I hope parents are paying attention for the sake of their kid's future health. While I'm not saying kids need to follow a strict ketogenic diet, more healthy fats and less processed food in their daily plan can go a long way. Life would have gone much more smoothly for me if I'd known all of this information when I was a teenager.

Back to our scheduled programming - my struggle with low blood pressure.

I seem to always go back to when I first began in the dieting world with many of my stories. I talk as if I can remember those days so vividly.

The sad truth is, I have far too many memories of attempting new diets because it was such a huge focus of my life starting at a young age. Thinking back to all of the girls I dieted alongside in high school, I know I'm not alone.

I have a friend from high school with whom I talked to daily about what we ate. That was the highlight of our day - listing all of the food we ate, while comparing and contrasting dieting notes. Sadly, she passed away from anorexia in her twenties. While that is an issue I never dealt with first hand, I witnessed her struggle. It was such a horrible existence.

If I can reach girls like that who are struggling with life so hardcore with my work, I'd love for them to know there is a better way.

I understand eating disorders like anorexia are mental disorders, but if these girls ate enough healthy fats to adequately fuel their brains instead of forcing more deprivation upon themselves, they might realize there is a healthier way to live when you eat foods that are right for you. These girls can thrive instead of using food, or lack of food, as a form of punishment. While I know this book won't change the world, if even one girl escapes the diet trap that so many fall into, then this is all worthwhile.

And now we're getting really deep. Let's bring focus back to my struggle with low blood pressure, and how I eventually found success with a ketogenic plan after taking steps to improve blood pressure.

Life with Low Blood Pressure

Whenever I attempted low carb plans in the past, I never understood low blood pressure played a part in my success or failure, or even with how I felt. The only thing I knew about blood pressure was when I visited the doctor, I received remarks from nurses like, "Wow, your blood pressure is great!" Then they blurted out numbers that meant nothing to me.

While I had no idea what they were talking about when they gave results like 90/65, I now understand that these numbers are far too low. The nurses viewed low numbers as a good thing because that's what they're taught. As long as your blood pressure isn't high, many view low blood pressure readings as healthy readings. How was I supposed to know low blood pressure could cause issues when I had so many nurses raving over my low readings?

I exhibited many of the problems that can come along with low blood pressure pretty much since I began my journey in the dieting world. I never connected the dots. While many of these health problems can have multiple causes, looking back at my history, I'm confident that several of my health issues stemmed from low blood pressure mixed with constant low calorie dieting that likely lowered my blood pressure even further.

Dating back even before high school, some of the health issues that can result from low blood pressure that I experienced include:

- Anxiety
- Depression
- Cravings
- Headaches
- Insomnia
- Fatigue

That pretty much runs the gamut of health issues that can arise from low blood pressure. I think the only one I'm missing is mental and emotional issues. After you hear the story of when my health was at its absolute worst, that might confirm that at some point, I hit them all.

A lot of teenage girls experience depression, and I was no exception. I had bouts of depression for decades. Since I was ashamed of feeling so sad, I never talked much about it.

Depression comes along with stigma in society. People who are depressed are seen as weak or mentally unstable. While I was a normal, functioning teen otherwise, I spent a good amount of time dealing with crying spells, and feeling hopeless and lonely, sometimes for no reason at all.

I had periods of depression like this throughout my mid-thirties. Even now, many people in my life still don't know about this struggle.

While I considered going on medication several times, that's not a route I ever took. I dealt with depression in private, and while it would come and go, the bouts of depression I experienced never improved to a level where I considered myself normal. Well, not at least until I stopped dieting and focussed more on balancing my body chemistry.

I also began to experience anxiety at an early age. You may not have guessed this about me since I'm writing a book where I'm spilling my deepest, darkest dieting secrets, but I tend to be a shy person in real life.

Well, at least I was shy. I'm pretty sure throughout high school there were other kids who questioned if I even talked. Back then, I had a pretty severe case of social anxiety.

Once I got into a room with people I felt comfortable with, I could talk and talk and talk; but if I was in a room with people I didn't know well, I'd freeze. My heart raced and I became a mime who smiled and laughed, but rarely talked.

I never thought balancing my body chemistry would help me overcome my shyness, but it's been a huge factor.

My anxiety did improve somewhat as I moved throughout the stages of life, like college and my first corporate job. Then I took a turn for the worse.

I experienced what was probably my biggest health crisis to date. While I just became accustomed to going through life with daily headaches, migraines that occasionally sent me to the ER, depression and all of the other symptoms I dealt with on a frequent basis, this next health crisis was the worst thing I've ever been through. It's one of those situations you'd never wish upon your worst enemy. Like, I don't even think Sansa Stark would wish this upon Ramsay Bolton, and that lady sat and watched as his dogs ate him alive.

Sorry, I had to lighten the mood a little … if you consider a story about a battered wife watching her husband being eaten alive by his dogs lightening the mood. Oh, and if you aren't caught up on *Game of Thrones*, sorry for the spoiler - but you're late to the party. Catch up already! It's a phenomenal show.

My Worst Health Crisis

Here's another spoiler alert. In the early 2000's, I had my first panic attack. At the time I didn't know what it was or how to get through it, but I basically felt like I was at death's door, and it came out of nowhere.

I remember when my first panic attack began. I was at the gym, running on the treadmill after work. While on the treadmill, my legs became a little itchy. By the time I arrived home and showered, I had red bumps all over, and I was itching like crazy.

I was fresh out of college, so I was living at home with my mom. I showed her the bumps and asked for her opinion. She thought it looked like an allergic reaction and told me if I felt short of breath, we needed to rush to the ER.

My first thought was my mom was being overly dramatic since this clearly was just a case of itchy skin. Itchy legs were definitely not drastic enough for an ambulance ride to the emergency room. I thought about what I might have eaten to pinpoint my reaction. My mom headed to the store to purchase Benadryl just in case.

In the time it took her to drive three blocks to Walgreens, my heart began racing and my throat tightened. I was never so scared in my life. As soon as she walked through the door, we rushed to the ER.

The support staff clearly had no idea what they were doing since they made me wait my turn in line. Did they not have eyes? How could they push me to the back of the waiting room while I was clearly dying right in front of them? I rocked back and forth like a crazy person, while grasping at my throat since I struggled to breathe.

When I finally saw a doctor, he asked a few questions and performed a few tests, but he couldn't tell me what was going on. He gave me an IV and allowed me to stay until I felt better. He told me to pay closer attention to what I eat in the event this happened again. He also sent me to an allergist for testing.

I visited both the allergist, as well as my regular doctor, to figure out what was going on. By the time I left both offices, I was prescribed nine new medications to deal with a problem neither could define.

Since they didn't know what was wrong with me, they stuck me on nine different prescription medications hoping one of them would do the trick. It was very similar to throwing darts at a dart board, while holding a beer in your other hand and balancing a cigarette in your mouth.

The allergist prescribed medications for asthma, which never made sense to me since I was in my 20's and never once had an asthma attack.

In fact, I ran on the treadmill many days without issue, so I couldn't comprehend an asthma diagnosis. Maybe asthmatics can run on treadmills without feeling out of breath. Since I never had asthma, I really had no clue. In the back of my mind, I felt like there had to be more to the story.

The anxiety I had about another allergic reaction like this happening again was awful.

One time I was prescribed penicillin for a sinus infection. I had too much anxiety to take it. Even though I had taken penicillin many times in my life, I feared all of the sudden I'd have an allergic reaction. I had a full on panic attack before I even swallowed the first pill. It took a good 30 minutes of staring at the pill and pacing the floors of my office in an attempt to calm myself down enough to take it.

This is how much of my life went at the time; constant anxiety over things that were just everyday events previously. The anxiety always built up and eventually led to another panic attack. The worst thing about the panic attacks I experienced is I didn't even know they were panic attacks because I was told I had asthma.

Luckily, on another visit to the allergist in my quest to fix what allied me, while reviewing my health history with a nurse, she flat out told me what I was experiencing sounded like panic attacks, not asthma.

This was a nurse at the allergist's office; the same doctor who took part in prescribing nine medications for health problems I didn't have, like asthma.

Thankfully my quest for knowledge about my own health began early on. I set out to research what was going on with my health and how I could fix it instead of relying on the advice of the doctors who told me I had asthma. This nurse was a blessing because I never would have thought to research panic attacks. I considered myself a normal, healthy girl and I associated panic attacks with mentally unstable people. I was only 22 at the time, which meant I was too young for mental problems, right?

As I sought out answers, I concluded I wasn't allergic to anything after all, as these were definitely full blown panic attacks.

I desperately wanted to go on a medication, like Zoloft, because I thought medication was the only answer. I basically would have taken anything to get out of the cycle of daily panic attacks. These panic attacks were so bad that I would have taken all of the asthma medications if that meant they'd stop. They truly were the worst thing I'd ever gone through in my life.

I'm so thankful my doctor didn't agree. He prescribed Zanax instead.

The funny part about my new prescription … I had too much anxiety to take Zanax, which is an anti anxiety medication. I figured anti anxiety pills would be the very thing that would make me stop breathing for good.

I kept the pills around just in case, but I never even took one pill. Finally understanding what was happening was enough to begin the healing process helped me take control of my life.

It took almost two years to recover from these horrible panic attacks. While I still dealt with anxiety for several years after the panic attacks stopped, regular old anxiety is a walk in the park compared to almost daily episodes where you feel like you're going to stop breathing at any moment for absolutely no reason at all.

More Low Blood Pressure Lows

I also started getting daily headaches around age ten. I visited several doctors to figure out the reason for the headaches. Even with extensive testing, including MRI's and blood tests, I never received many answers. I did have one doctor who advised that I should switch my diet since what I ate could have been a factor.

Attempting to talk a teenager into a better diet is a tough task. While I was already deep into diet mentality at the time, I couldn't bear to give up some of the foods the doctor suggested.

Looking back, I applaud this doctor for trying to help me with better food choices. At the time I thought he was nuts, but now I realize he was onto something. At the time there weren't very many doctors who would advise you to change how you eat over prescribing a medication to improve headaches.

Since it was the 90's, he advised a low fat plan with more fruit and whole grains, combined with diet products like diet soda and sugar free products. While not what I'd consider great advice knowing what I now know, at least he was sort of on the right track. Back then, that's pretty much what everyone meant when they told you to eat better - fat free and sugar-free. In other words, carbs and chemical laden diet products.

The headaches continued almost daily through my mid-thirties. At some point, they shifted from annoying headaches where I popped a few Advil to keep them under control, to extremely painful migraines, which at times sent me to the ER due to intense pain. There were even times I was sure I was having a brain aneurysm.

Of course, I always had strong cravings for junk food whenever I tried to go on any diet.

As I talked about in the previous chapter, the cravings for carbs like crackers and bread not only were strong because I missed the crunch, but they became a necessity because the nausea I felt on low carb plans became so intense that I thought my body required these carbs just to function.

I also experienced insomnia and fatigue for large chunks of my life. The fatigue I chalked up to either the daily headaches, because daily headaches tend to zap your energy, or to the fact that I was a busy teenager who worked hard for good grades, typically worked at least one after school job, and also participated in after school activities. Not hard to determine that fatigue could result from a schedule like that.

I had nothing to attribute the insomnia. With the schedule I just described, surely I'd be exhausted and need rest, right?

Nope.

I spent far too many nights tossing and turning, trying everything I could to fall asleep. There were so many nights that I'd go to bed around 10 pm, and I wouldn't fall asleep until 2 or 3 am, which was just a few hours before my alarm went off to start the day.

While I woke up feeling exhausted most days, I had things to accomplish to be successful in life, so I always pushed through.

This type of sleeping schedule persisted on and off from the time I was a teenager through my mid-thirties. I had nights where I struggled to fall asleep. I also had many other nights where I'd fall asleep easily, but then an hour or two into slumber something would awaken me, and it would take hours of tossing and turning before I got back to sleep.

I even went through a period where I relied on over the counter sleeping pills to help me stay asleep. I started taking sleeping pills on and off throughout high school, but even then I knew they weren't great for my overall health, so I stopped.

I picked the habit up again in my early 20's when my panic attacks began. Forcing sleep was the only way to escape the attacks that were common at night. At the time there were many nights I truly believed once I fell asleep, I most likely wouldn't wake up. That's how life consuming panic attacks are.

As I previously mentioned, I exhibited all of these symptoms of low blood pressure on and off for decades. My doctors always told me my blood pressure was great, so how was I to know that the way I was eating - mostly low calorie, and at times both low calorie and low carb, had anything to do with all of these chronic health problems I experienced for so long?

Many incorrectly assume if you're overweight, then your blood pressure must be high.

Most of these same people still follow the outdated advice to give up salt because the media scares us into believing too much salt will result in a heart attack. They give up salt without ever checking where their blood pressure is on a daily basis.

Thankfully with keto becoming more mainstream, people are fearing salt less, and are adding more high quality sea salt to food. While many in the keto world are coming around to salt, I feel like a lot of them are just following the crowd and may not fully understand why they're all of the sudden so salt happy.

So whether blood pressure is too high or too low, our keto friends add salt. Some ketoers also don't always understand that salting your food, or supplementing with a high quality salt in other forms, isn't the only step many need in order to raise blood pressure for the long haul.

They also may not understand that when they do supplement with salt, especially at the beginning, that a few dashes of salt here and there won't cut it. Some may need to supplement with all the salt!

When I went into low carb plans in the past - you know, all of those times I miserably failed low carb diets, I had low blood pressure. Even though at every doctor visit the nurses beamed about readings, it was far too low to function as a normal human being should. This made following a low carb plan far more difficult than it needs to be since dropping carbs even further can drop blood pressure even lower.

Looking back at all of the symptoms I experienced throughout my twenty year diet history, some merely annoying, while some were life altering, all signs point to low blood pressure.

Sure, there were other things going on with my chemistry that played a part, but once I learned why keeping blood pressure in a normal range is important, and then I followed through with the steps to improve my blood pressure, most of these health issues vanished. Hopefully you can see how I'm connecting the dots.

Keto and Low Blood Pressure Don't Mix

Everytime I attempted low carb plans before becoming educated about how to succeed on a low carb plan with my newfound info, I always went into them with a typical dieter's mindset. I rushed into these plans without allowing my body time to adjust. I just wanted the weight to fall off as quickly as possible so I could bring junk carbs back into my life. The harder I pursued a low carb plan, the happier I'd be when it was done and over with.

Except, my struggle was never done and over with.

I may have lost a few pounds, or sometimes even more than just a few, but I could never see a low carb plan through to my goal. Then I'd beat myself up over failing yet another low carb diet. Then I'd get back to strict calorie counting and over exercising. Again.

I'm sure if you've fallen into this type of low carb cycle, then you know cravings for carbs can become intense. Every thought revolves around food, especially the food you're depriving yourself of.

If your blood pressure is low prior to cutting carbs, it likely will go even lower once you slash carb intake to a low carb or keto level. This is the perfect storm for diet disaster.

Not only will the food you 'can't eat' constantly be on your mind, but once your blood pressure drops low enough, you'll cave and eat all of the carbs you've been obsessing over for weeks.

Then you blame yourself, even though it's not really your fault.

Your physiology drove your body to scream out for carbs since your body isn't able to function appropriately off of the fuel you're providing. Your body views this as a life or death situation, even if that's not the truth. If you never take the time to work with your body by improving low blood pressure, you will continue to follow this cycle. This will continue to happen no matter how strong willed you think you'll be when it comes to sticking to your plan this time around.

When I finally became educated about the role of blood pressure on a low carb plan, I went to Target and purchased a blood pressure monitor in order to test at home. It wasn't expensive - probably less than $30, and it's been so worth having this information about myself to help guide me in the right direction for success.

When I first began testing, my blood pressure averaged somewhere around 90/60 on a good day. This was my blood pressure while lying down in a calm state at least two hours after a meal.

If you only rely on blood pressure readings you get at the doctor's office, those are usually artificially inflated readings. If you happened to have just eaten right before your visit, your reading is definitely inflated.

Measuring blood pressure at home under the right circumstances is the way you can receive accurate results. This simple step can help you understand how much effort you need to put into raising blood pressure on your keto plan; or if you should even follow keto in the first place.

Here's a hint - if your blood pressure is consistently low two hours after meals, you may need to do more work to balance your body chemistry before you'll find success on keto.

If you're still unsure how to properly measure blood pressure, check out the digestion course to watch videos that walk you through this step. Learning this basic info about yourself can really make or break your keto success.

This is one of the reasons I'm thankful I didn't even know about keto when I began a low carb plan. Had I known about the amazing results people were getting on keto, I may have forced a diet that wasn't right for my physiology.

By the time I learned about keto, I was already an entire year into working on improving aspects of my chemistry, like blood pressure, which made following keto so much easier. I found a lot of success once my body was properly balanced.

Just to be clear, while I say I never knew what keto was previously, I have tried plans I found in magazines referred to as "Atkins Supercharged." Looking back, those plans were basically keto plans. This means I did try keto before I fixed myself up, and I failed miserably each time.

You gotta fix that blood pressure!

My Transition to Keto Success

I keep going on and on about how I improved digestion and balanced chemistry in order to find success with keto. I'm sure you're wondering exactly what this means. I didn't really understand the value at the time, but instead of rushing into a very low carb, high fat plan, I allowed my body time to adjust as it was ready.

At the very beginning, I was still eating somewhere around 150 grams of carbs per day. While you may scream in terror at that number if you've been struggling to survive on only 20 carbs each day, it's still about half of what most people consume on a S.A.D. plan.

Since prior to restarting my low carb routine I was all about living my best SAD life, I still saw progress just by lowering my diet to 150 carbs. Back then, the days I ate less than 100 carbs in a day were days I felt proud.

Once I cut carbs low enough to constitute a low carb plan, I started adding coconut oil to meals in order to help my body learn how to digest fat better. I also added salt when I could, but not directly to coconut oil because that's probably gross.

After years of being told salt would kill me, I trained my body not to really love salt. Sure, I was accustomed to processed junk filled with sodium, and while that will inflate blood pressure, it's not the same thing. I had to relearn how to add high quality salt to food whenever I could.

I also tried tricks like adding salt to water, but that definitely wasn't my favorite. I couldn't take all in one mineral supplements, like Concentrace Mineral Drops, because my body chemistry just wasn't having it. Since I commonly leaned catabolic, this meant I had to limit magnesium in order to feel like a human.

If you don't know this about yourself, and you randomly follow the keto crowd without testing your chemistry, you could be loading up on all the magnesium since that's the common keto wisdom being dispensed.

Many chronic dieters make their way into a keto plan with this imbalance, and they don't even know it. Once you add magnesium into the mix, especially at night as is also commonly advised, you will feel like you're falling apart, and you'll have no clue why you feel so bad.

Take the time to learn this stuff and test yourself. It's really worth it. Don't you make me link that digestion course again.

I spent a good year weaning myself off carbs. This time around, I was smart. Instead of jumping from a diet filled to the brim with processed foods straight to a plan that's 100% real food, I took my time to allow my body to catch up with my brain.

Sure, low-to-medium glycemic index carbs that are real food will always help you get the quickest progress, but if I jumped right from all of the processed junk I subsisted on up until this point, I would have failed.

Been there, done that too many times to count.

I started slowly with 'healthier' processed choices, and while healthier than the trans fats laden junk I previously mistook as food, moving away from consuming even 'healthy' processed food over time allowed the stable weight I enjoy today.

I recommend taking time to transition if you need this, but be sure to keep your eye on the prize and ultimately shoot for a diet filled with real food as your final destination.

Don't continue to mistake processed foods as an appropriate fuel source for too long. For improved health and faster progress, understand even 'healthier' versions of processed food should only be a stepping stone to your ultimate goal.

Also understand that rushing to reach your ultimate goal, be it a diet filled with real food, or even dropping a size or two by next week, isn't doing you any favors when it comes to progress. Allow yourself adequate time to make the transition to real food, as well as hitting bigger weight loss milestones.

Beyond salting my food with high quality salts and lowering carb intake over time, while still keeping carbs high enough to keep blood pressure in a normal range, I also took Beatine HCL with most meals.

HCL, which stands for hydrochloric acid (aka stomach acid) works with your body to properly break down the nutrients you eat into usable sources. If you've spent years following low protein diets, or taking medications like antacids which destroy stomach acid production, your body will view the protein you eat as toxins and store it in fat cells.

Supplementing with HCL was an important step for me to find long term success. If you have chronic low blood pressure, this is a step you need to consider.

If you fall into this low blood pressure category, simply over salting your food won't be enough for long term success. You need to help your body out with proper food digestion after years of screwing up your body with inappropriate food choices or too many medications used overtime.

I also stopped exercising at obsessively high levels of cardio. Instead of spending 60-90 minutes each day performing intense elliptical sessions, I focussed more on walking 3-4 days each week. I also tried harder to incorporate resistance training into my week. Working out with weights has never been my favorite part of exercise, even though I know these workouts are really important for improved health. I do my best to keep it in the mix.

Once I followed most of these steps for about a year, I lost somewhere around 70 pounds. Of course when you're in the thick of hitting your ultimate goal, it seems like the pounds never melt off fast enough. Now I can look back and realize losing 70 pounds in a year is amazing progress … and that amazing progress was all thanks to low carb and improved digestion.

I wanted to point this out so you'll realize that you don't necessarily need to follow a strict keto plan to find success. Working towards improved chemistry and digestion, while also continuing to lower carbs over time, can lead to a ton of success - as it did for me!

Easing into a low carb plan like this also helped establish low carb as a lifestyle. I no longer dream of the day I can add back all of my favorite junk carbs. That doesn't mean I don't occasionally indulge, because there are times I do, but I no longer plan to indulge like that on a daily basis.

After maintaining what I lost for more than three years, I'm confident the 100+ pounds I lost are finally gone for good. I also feel like a human while living my low carb lifestyle since my blood pressure has finally normalized. I no longer have to pour massive amounts of salt on my meals. There are some days I use very little salt at all, yet my body stays balanced.

Of course all of the health problems I described earlier in this chapter are also long gone. It's such a blessing to no longer deal with bouts of depression and constant anxiety. I no longer experience intense carb cravings, and I finally get a good night's sleep most nights . While I still have occasional sleep interruptions, those mostly come in the form of a 5 year old who's scared of the monsters hiding under his bed.

I also haven't had a migraine since 2015. If you've ever experienced migraines, I know you understand how absolutely life changing this is. Living my life migraine free is probably the biggest victory I've had from putting in the work to improve digestion, and that's saying a lot since I've experienced so many health wins.

I no longer struggle just to feel like a human, and I keep the weight I lost off with ease. I'm so blessed I no longer have to deal with chronic health problems that destroyed the quality of my life for so long.

If you still believe blood pressure is just a number doctor's monitor to make sure you're not in stroke territory, now you understand there's way more to the story!

Chapter 7: Not Pooping Isn't Fun and Other Things I Discovered About Low Stomach Acid

Since we've been together for a few chapters, and we've gotten to know a bit about each other, let's talk poop! If you felt like you knew me before reaching this chapter, we're about to become BFF's on a whole new level.

Buckle up and grab a few tissues; shit's about to get real. That tissue might come in handy if you laugh a little too hard at my misfortune, or maybe you'll need it to cover your eyes in terror. This chapter could really go either way.

Just as I have plenty of stories about my impaired ability to digest fat, and we talked all about how I displayed pretty much every symptom there is when it comes to low blood pressure, I also found myself struggling to digest protein after years of abusing my body in the low calorie, yo-yo dieting world.

Shocker!

Thankfully my protein saga isn't quite as long as my other stories, but if you attempt a keto diet with poor stomach acid production, this chapter might be the most important yet. Don't skip it because I used a fancy term like stomach acid production and you don't think it applies. Trust me, I never thought it applied to me either.

Since it's estimated at least 5 out of every 10 people have low stomach acid, it's important for all of those people to learn how they too can help their bodies improve this major digestive malfunction. Also, 5 out of every 10 is just a low guestimate, as it's likely closer to 9 out of every 10.

I hope those 9 out of every 10 people find this book so they can get help for their low stomach acid! Since you stumbled upon this life altering information, do your part and let at least 10 people know about this book. With so many people that have low stomach acid, you'll be doing a solid for many of the people you encounter.

While there are some who can successfully follow a keto plan and never even have a second thought about protein, there are others who are so insulin sensitive that if they even look at one extra ounce of protein, it immediately converts into sugar and kicks them out of ketosis!

That gluconeogenesis can really sneak up on ya'll!

Ha. I just said ya'll like I'm southern.

Born and raised Chicago girl here. Chicagoans don't say ya'll, although I do have quite a few aunts that say you's, as in, "I love you's," or "You's guys need need more melk."

Alright you's guys, let's get back to protein and how I figured out protein and I were no longer on speaking terms … at least for a period of time.

Symptoms of low stomach acid include:

- Constipation
- Heartburn
- Reflux
- Low blood pressure
- Burping
- Bloating
- Nausea

Check, check, check, check, check, check and check.

I already mentioned the first time I read *Kick Your Fat in the Nuts*, I was pretty sure I was somehow the muse. Throughout my twenty year yo-yo diet history, I displayed every single one of these problems.

Some of them were obvious to me - like the heartburn that woke me up from a dead sleep, while clutching my chest in pain, as well as the not so pleasant nausea I felt, especially after eating a big steak.

Other symptoms weren't quite as obvious because I either didn't know to look for them, had no idea they were affecting me, or that they had anything to do with digesting what I ate.

I already told you my story of woe that is low blood pressure. I had all of those signs as well, but never knew my blood pressure was low since doctors and nurses always gave two thumbs up when I got readings like 90/60. Still, they had zero answers when I asked the reasons I experienced bouts of depression and I had constant anxiety.

Funny, isn't it?

Well, not ha ha funny. I was depressed and not laughing at anything. More funny in the sense that depression and anxiety are deemed medical problems, yet everytime I brought it up, the medical community either wanted to shove me on a medication to temporarily mask symptoms, or dole me out to another doctor to talk through my feelings.

The thing about depression - you don't feel like yourself, and you don't really feel up to talking to anyone, littlelone a stranger you've never met. I never took the therapy route.

Wait, I take that back. I actually did take the therapy route one time in college when my first real boyfriend left me for some floozy he met in his nutrition class. How's that for irony? I bet she doesn't have four health and nutrition books on Amazon.

When I first learned of said floozy, I was so heart broken that I could barely pry myself out of bed. The devastation was real. Since the school year just kicked off and I needed to get back to some semblance of a normal life, I made an appointment with the school's free student therapist.

During my first appointment, I barely spoke a word. It didn't matter since any words that managed to slip through my lips were immediately drowned out by my wailing sobs of grief. I couldn't stop the flood of tears, no matter how hard I tried. As humiliating as it was to express the depths of my despair in front of a therapist who only showed up to score class credit, I had zero control.

That first week post break up, the mere mention of my ex sent a rainstorm of tears. And it didn't stop at tears. My involuntary reaction was something straight out of an 80's John Hughes flick. All I can remember was how the thick snot dripping from my nose made it impossible to breathe, and that my chest was so heavy that I really would have appreciated a little assistance removing the elephant that was apparently stomping all over my chest. That's how hard I cried.

I hit up the student therapist again the next week, but this time I was perfectly fine. Seriously, not even a single tear was shed. I actually spent the session laughing.

Needless to say our student therapist was shocked at the difference a week made. I think it had a little something to do with a quick trip I took earlier that week to the ex's house to drop off some stuff he left in my dorm.

When I arrived, he answered the door in his brand new birthday outfit from the floozy.

He straight up resembled Freddy Mercury post Live Aid, which would have been OK if we were still circa 1975. Problem was, in the early 2000's this outfit was just too much since no one I was aware of donned netted tanks and pleather pants. At least not men anyway. Especially not men who spent their lives in the gym obsessing over perfect biceps.

And he was that guy who spent all day obsessing over perfect biceps in the gym. Apparently he spent his nights obsessing over his fly moves at Studio 54. I definitely wasn't aware of this secret life in the five years we were together, so I suppose the floozy allowed him to shine.

I actually found his exact outfit online. I don't think I'm allowed to add the photo to this book, but click here if you're curious. And if you click through the link, imagine that outfit on a 6'2, 220 lb bodybuilder type of guy. Once the tears stop, come back to read more.

Needless to say, I moved on with my life and never looked back. I also never went back to therapy. I'm definitely not saying there's anything wrong with therapy, but ever since I took time to improve digestion, I just don't have the need.

Since uncontrollable tears relate more to low blood pressure, let's get back to protein and how I had no clue my body wasn't breaking protein down very well.

While I experienced burping with most meals, they were polite burps … not the big ole' belches most 4 year olds find hilarious. I couldn't even conjure up a belch like that if I tried, and I thought the tiny, quiet burps were just a part of life. So of course I had no idea those were a sign of anything askew, especially when it came to the delicious steak dinner I just devoured.

As far as bloating, while I've always heard women talk about being bloated, I had no idea what they meant. I knew my clothing felt tighter throughout the day, especially around my waist, but I just chalked that up the instant weight gain I experienced the second I ate pretty much anything.

Back then I was stuck in a continuous cycle of constant weight loss or weight regain, so feeling chubby in my wardrobe was just part of life. I had no idea there was an actual term for my pants choking my belly button with marshmallowy fluff hanging over the sides by the end of the day.

And what about constipation?

While this was the biggest problem I dealt with when it comes to low stomach acid, at the time I had no clue. When people talked about severe constipation, they were talking about me, and I was oblivious.

I bet you at least chucked at that thought. How can someone have chronic constipation and not even know it? We eat, we poop, we eat, we poop … and if you don't follow a similar pattern, you're constipated. We all know this, right?

But do we all know this? Because I had no clue.

I never knew it's actually normal to poop every single day since prior to improving digestion, I never even came close. Back then, I was lucky if I pooped once a week.

With my body busy storing so much of what I ate as toxins instead of eliminating them daily via bowel movements, it's no wonder I struggled with weight loss for so many years. Still, I had zero clue I was constipated.

I incorrectly assumed that you were only considered constipated if you felt physically bad from your lack of potty time, or if when you felt like you had to go, you sat on the toilet for hours straining, unable to squeeze anything out.

When I did my duty once each week, I was in and out of the bathroom in between commercials, and then I moved on with my life. I never felt bad or like I was missing something, so the fact that I was constipated never crossed my mind.

The True Meaning of Constipation

I finally learned the true meaning of constipation after I had my first son. I had a C-section, and even though the nurses began a stool softener protocol day one post pregnancy, I didn't poop for days. Since this was nothing new, I didn't think it was an issue. Turns out my naive train of thought, a la Vivian in *Pretty Woman*, was a big mistake. HUGE!

The nurses asked several times each day if I had my first post pregnancy bowel movement. I spent five days in the hospital recovering from my C-section, and they refused to release me until after the first post pregnancy BM.

Some time around day four, it happened. While it wasn't exactly comfortable, nothing was comfortable four days after being cut in half to have my tiny bundle of joy ripped from my womb. I couldn't figure out why the nurses made such a big deal about pooping; at least not until a few days later.

Thankfully my mom was there to help me care for said bundle of joy when this next event happened … otherwise I'm not quite sure how I would have made it through this ordeal with a brand new bundle who required constant care.

Even though I followed doctor's orders and dosed up appropriately on the stool softeners sent home with me, these stool softeners did nothing to save me from the trauma about to unfold. Nothing!

A few days into living up the comfort of my own home, I felt like I had to go. It instinctively felt like it might take a minute, so I made sure my mom had the baby covered. I waltzed into the bathroom with no clue about the pain on the horizon.

One hour.

I was hunched over the toilet for one hour straining to push out whatever demon lay dormant inside me. While I was previously warned not to strain while doing the deed since that could result in the 'roids, straining during this, um, we'll call it 'the incident,' was inevitable.

Seriously, I just had a 7 lb, 9 oz baby cut from my insides a few days prior, and that had nothing on the pain I felt trying to push out that first real bowel movement post C-section. I was in the bathroom for at least thirty minutes prior to experiencing even a hint of progress.

The pain was excruciating. I could barely focus on the task at hand because there was so much pain. And then I panicked.

While ensuring baby care was covered, I didn't even think to bring my phone into the bathroom with me. It was at this point it dawned on me there was at least a slight chance I'd have to call 9-1-1 to have the other half of me cut open for some sort of relief.

I know you think I'm being overly dramatic since maybe you've noticed I have a minor flair for drama at times ... like a few sentences ago when I casually mentioned being cut in half to have a baby ripped from my insides, but I'm dead serious this time.

I strained so hard and for so long that I actually feared the poop would have to be surgically removed. It felt like I was attempting to release a ten pound bowling ball from an area that has no business housing a ten pound bowling ball.

That first real post C-section poop is scary, to say the least. I know this to be true, as it was not an isolated event. I had to go through this trauma again after baby #2. Even when you think you're prepared, there's just no way to prepare for this kind of stress.

I apologize to any men reading this. I understand you're horrified, but if you have a wife who bore your baby, especially if it was a C-section birth, go hug her. Drop whatever you're doing and give her a big squeeze. This woman went through birth twice, and she only has one baby to show for it.

If you don't have a wife, at the very least go tell your mother how much you love her. Show a woman who had to endure this life altering mega poop some love. We deserve it.

My entire point of this dramatic tale is I finally figured out the true meaning of constipation. I also figured out my husband had something called poop sticks that he sometimes used when his BM's were too big to flush.

While pre-birth (the poop, not the kid), I never even dreamed of letting my husband in on the fact that I even went number two, I had no choice but to call in reinforcements to get that monster down the pipes. As someone who suffered from constipation for most of her life, I didn't even know poop sticks were a thing, or that he used them.

Seriously, I just had this man's baby and it's like I barely knew him at all.

I hope you're LOLing right about now instead of gasping in horror because a lady dared talk poop. For those covering your eyes in horror, that's not an efficient way to read a book. Since I'm all about efficiency, let's move on.

Constipation Is More than Mega Poops

It was six months after 'the incident' that I read *Kick Your Fat in the Nuts*. I learned that while 'the incident' is definitely considered constipation, it's not the only way to experience constipation. There are several other ways you can experience constipation, and this includes those of us who only poop once each week.

Who knew? Definitely not me!

While perhaps that's a very obvious case of constipation, prior to finding this info no one ever told me that I was supposed to poop everyday, so I just didn't know. Plus, as shy as I was, poop talk was definitely far from the list of conversations I felt comfortable having with anyone else.

Check out that shy girl now! Here I am telling anyone who will listen about the time I had to take a dump the size of my dog.

Yep, that's my life's purpose - this glorious path to help others by talking mega dumps and poop sticks.

More Symptoms of Low Stomach Acid

Even though I experienced so many symptoms of not digesting protein well throughout my life, and even though I visited many doctors to help improve some of these health issues, I never once came across a permanent solution.

Think back to the last chapter where I talked about my worst health crisis to date. You'll recall that at one point I was on nine different medications after I had what I thought was an allergic reaction. One of those nine medications was Nexium.

This is an acid reducer for the chronic heartburn I experienced. Before graduating to the prescription stuff, I took full advantage of over the counter solutions, like Tums. Before Tums became a necessity, a glass of milk helped settle the burn. Basically, for as long as I can remember, heartburn has been an active part of my life.

Even though I wasn't happy about taking nine prescriptions on the daily, Nexium was a necessity since heartburn was an everyday event. Plus, I had a few family members who suffered from heartburn so severe that they were told by doctors it would eventually develop into esophageal cancer if they didn't reduce acid with prescriptions. We were all told this condition was hereditary, so I didn't want to take any chances by skipping this med.

Even though esophageal cancer typically affects our elders, like those in their 70's, 80's and 90's, and I was only twenty something at the time, I didn't want to develop this hereditary death sentence at an earlier than expected age, so I needed that prescription!

Uneducated I was. So uneducated I was. Don't even get me started on those doctors!

As I weaned off many of the nine prescriptions, with my doctor's approval and guidance, I stayed on acid reducers for years. When Nexium no longer worked, I switched to Prilosec, and I continued to follow a pattern of adding the next biggest and baddest acid reducer for years. I was in my twenties!

Even with upgrades in prescriptions over time, there were many days I had to pop a few supplemental Tums. They were fruity and didn't taste too bad, so I never really minded this addition, especially since they provided relief from the burning.

To go along with heartburn, I also had reflux. Nearly every meal I ate was followed up with acid shooting right back up my throat, followed by round two of the meal I ate thirty minutes prior.

If re-indulging in the meal you just ate sounds pleasant to you, I can assure you it's nothing of the sort. And while not pleasant in the least, I thought this happened to everyone. I popped another Tums to ease the burning and called it a success. Why I thought choking up your meal thirty minutes later was normal is beyond me. I guess when something happens so frequently, and no one is there to tell you differently, you just assume it's something that happens to everyone.

When I became pregnant with my first son, heartburn became life. Thankfully Tums was one of the few medications on the pregnancy approved list, because man did I pop those tablets. Once I got sick of the fruity Tums, I switched over to the peppermint Tums. Once I could no longer stand even the thought of another one of those, I just had to grin it, bear it, and choke down another chalky tablet to get through an esophagus lit ablaze.

Where Did All The Stomach Acid Go?

If you're already properly educated on all things digestion, you know I received pretty bad info when it comes to heartburn relief. Hearing these stories about how I destroyed any lingering stomach acid I had is probably even making you angry. Maybe you're throwing your half empty bottle of Tums at this book.

Trust me, I get it. All of the bad info I was given by trusted, supposedly well-trained sources over the years makes me angry too.

Popping antacids isn't the only way I completely obliterated my stomach acid overtime. All of those years spent following low calorie diets made up of low fat foods like pasta, breads, and other processed foods definitely played its part.

What I did not focus on all of those years were the real foods my body needed to thrive. When I swapped out diet convenience foods instead of eating real food options, like steak and chicken beyond the processed chunks found on top of a Lean Cuisine, this aided in the destruction of my stomach acid.

You don't need a lot of stomach acid to break down a big plate of pasta, or a sandwich with a few pieces of lunch meat, but that's really mostly bread. When your stomach acid isn't being called upon on a regular basis like it should be when you eat a diet made up of real food, your body produces less stomach acid.

Let me point out that yes, I use big phrases like, "destruction of my stomach acid," or "I completely destroyed my stomach acid," but hopefully you know that's just my flair for drama. What I really mean by all of this is my body began producing less stomach acid since I no longer needed to produce as much with the processed foods that don't contain much protein.

This doesn't even mention all of the acid reducers I took over time did their job; they reduced my stomach acid, just as their descriptions imply.

Whenever I attempted real food based diets filled with meat, those diets didn't go so well for me. When starting these plans, I experienced nausea, especially upon eating meat, and the cravings I had for processed carbs were intense.

My body didn't have what it took to break down the real food that real food diets required, so it instead cried out for the processed foods it had the ability to break down for fuel. I was usually able to white knuckle my way through some of these diets for at least a little while, but it was never long before I found myself face first in a box of crackers to settle the nausea.

After shoving down every last Tums sold in the tri-state area during pregnancy, I experienced a new low when it came to eating meat. Pre-pregnancy, steak was one of my favorite foods. Soon after I had my baby, my family met up for a holiday meal at a steakhouse; one of those really fancy ones with thick cuts of steak where everyone shares huge sides.

This exhausted mama was ready to eat every last one her sleep deprived feelings with a big ole' New York Strip. Except when I ordered the steak, it tasted like a dead cow.

I mean, I understand that's essentially what steak is, but it always tasted like a delicious meal previously. I ordered my hunk of meat medium-well, so I couldn't understand why I could only manage a few bites of one of my favorite meals in the whole world.

I did have a similar experience with meat early on in pregnancy where all red meat tasted raw, and I couldn't eat it for at least 3-4 months. Since I had the baby three months prior by this point, and there was no way I was pregnant again, I couldn't figure out what was going on.

It was a mystery to me; a sad and unfortunate mystery ... at least until I learned about all of the awful things I put my body through for more than twenty years with the constant popping of acid reducers, as well as other medications that merely masked health symptoms. Focussing on processed foods like 'healthy' whole grains and processed carbs also didn't do me any favors when it came to digestive health.

Then, and only then, the dead cow steak incident made sense.

How I Improved Stomach Acid Production

Once I determined that I checked all of the boxes of low stomach acid, I began taking steps to help my body improve production. While nervous to start the supplement routine, I implemented Beet Flow and HCL into my routine right away. Just as with many others who explore this routine, I figured I'd have to take these supplements for a month, maybe two tops, and then decades of damage would be magically reversed.

I know that's the way so many of us think about improving years of health problems - like it should be an overnight fix. When I see it in writing, I can see how silly that statement is. I spent decades destroying my stomach acid production, and I expected to reverse all of the damage in a month, two tops.

That's right up there with everyone who spent years gaining weight, and once they determine they're ready to lose it, many expect huge losses each week so they can hit their goal weight by summer, which happens to be less than three months away.

Friends, life doesn't work that way.

I started with Beet Flow to get sludgy bile moving, since I also checked most categories for sludgy bile flow. After a few days on Beet Flow, I was extremely nervous to take that first HCL pill, mostly because I didn't know what would happen after it slid down the hatch.

Before popping that first pill, several questions anxiously ran through my mind:

Would it rush right through me, resulting in explosive diarrhea?

Would it tragically become lodged in my throat and burn the entire way down?

Could I die from taking a natural supplement?

In the perfect catch 22, I needed this supplement to reverse years of anxiety, but taking any new supplement became a chore because I had so much anxiety! This was especially true with a supplement that had the word acid in the name. While popping acid pills trudged up a whole new level of anxiety, I wanted to lose weight and nothing else got my scale to budge, so I took a deep breath, closed my eyes, and swallowed the capsule.

And … I was fine.

I made it to the recommended dosage of five pills per meal without too much drama. In fact, the only issue I noticed with five HCLs per meal was at times I had increased heartburn.

I learned in the support group that this likely meant I needed a round of D-Limonene to help with bacterial overgrowth. Being that I was also testing my chemistry and I leaned way catabolic, I could only take D-Limonene early in the morning and every other day to avoid pushing myself even further catabolic.

There was nothing scary about D-Limonene. I did experience orange flavored burps on the days I took those, but I didn't really mind burping up orange flavor. Orange flavored burps were a walk in the park compared to the fish burps I experienced during pregnancy when I was told to take fish oil supplements. Coming from a girl who can't stand even the smell of fish, I'll take orange flavored burps over fish burps any day of the week.

Once I got through a round of D-Limonene, I was able to add HCL back into the mix without incident. Was it a pain in the butt popping nine supplement pills with most meals?

At first, yes. The routine I followed was 1 Bio-C, 2 Beet Flow, 1 Digestizyme and 5 HCL's with most meals. No one really wants to take that many pills with meals, I get it. So while popping supplements with meals wasn't my favorite part of the program, I pulled up my big girl pants and I dealt with it.

After a few weeks, taking supplements with meals just became a habit. In fact, if I ever went out for a meal where I forgot to bring supplements with me, I kind of felt naked without them. At least my meal felt naked without them; I promise I remained fully clothed.

While I didn't notice a huge difference on days I did take them, I mean beyond not having, "Oh my God, I have to sit down because this heartburn is going to kill me," kind of pain, on the days I forgot to bring supplements with me, I noticed a big difference. My meals felt heavier and I didn't have as much energy later that day.

Over time I noticed big changes to the way I felt as well. I wasn't getting sick nearly as often as I had in the past. The heartburn was finally gone, and I was pooping at least on an every other day basis.! That's a huge change that eventually got even better.

In fact, one of the tricks I used to lose weight when I first started was a handwritten food journal. One of the things I kept track of in the journal was the days I pooped. I can't tell you how excited I was the very first week I was able to write down that I pooped every single day.

It's the little wins, people!

I also previously took St John's Wort pretty regularly for anxiety. Even with the kind that claimed prescription strength on the bottle, my anxiety was off the charts most days. Once my body was better at breaking down the food I ate, my blood pressure normalized and I no longer felt constant anxiety. Depression cleared up as well.

By the time I stumbled across a keto diet, I still recall first reading about keto flu. Most articles suggested taking all the magnesium and sea salt supplements to not only get through keto flu, but to succeed on keto long term.

When beginning keto, I didn't take very much magnesium since it wasn't right for my chemistry that I was still working on balancing. I did add more sea salt, which helped take me through the keto flu stage, but I didn't really need to load up on it as much as everyone else urges. That's actually a great thing for me since I gagged every time I attempted to place a quarter teaspoon of salt under my tongue. I also prefer water very plain, so adding a lot of salt to water throughout the day wasn't desirable either.

As I said earlier in this chapter, I thought I could add these supplements in for a month or two, and solve all of the stomach acid problems I spent decades creating. That's a big NO for me. I followed the supplement routine for about a year before I really thought I improved stomach acid enough to wean myself off HCL. It came at a good time too. Just as I weaned myself off HCL, I became pregnant with baby #2.

While I didn't take supplements during pregnancy, I did have a relapse with Tums. I wasn't sure at the time if that was the right step to take while pregnant, but the heartburn was so intense that just adding a little acid with apple cider vinegar wasn't cutting it. This means I got back to the supplement routine after baby #2 was born. This time, of course, I knew exactly what to do.

Not only did I feel better with this new routine, but I was finally able to lose weight with a low carb plan. Then, I was able to supercharge that weight loss once I switched over to a keto plan. Not only did I lose weight, but it was a much easier process when my body felt nourished by the food I ate when I had the ability to break it down. My stomach no longer felt heavy after meals, and the intense carb cravings I felt while on low carb plans in the past vanished.

Sure, no one wants to take supplements to help improve health, but if you're showing the signs I mentioned when it comes to poor protein digestion, it is so worth further research to figure out if these steps will help you.

When I went into this plan, I had to have faith that it would work for me since nothing else worked at the time. If you decide this is the same path you need to follow for low carb or keto success, hopefully you've mustered up the faith that these steps will work for you.

Luckily, you also have my experience to learn from. Reading my story and knowing what I experienced along the way can better illustrate the steps you may need to take, and what you can expect.

Chapter 8: You Big Fat Keto Cheater

Keto is a surprisingly easy plan to follow, yet so many make it far too complicated!

I want to take this next section to explain my view on one of the most controversial topics keto has to offer. This is probably the most confusing part of keto, and the reason many fail to find success; you know, beyond the controversy of eating low fat on a high fat diet.

I'm eight chapters in, and I still can't quite figure that one out.

There are many opinions, and much confusion, in the ketosphere when it comes to *how* to count the carbs you eat. Since it's vital for some ketoers to limit carbs to less than 20 per day for keto success, I'd say it's important to make sure you're counting carbs correctly, while getting the most out of the carbs you choose.

I'm about to ask you to close your eyes.

Now obviously your eyes need to be open in order to read this book, so let's just pretend. This is especially true if you're reading this while on the treadmill. Let's be smart about this!

While being fueled by ketones may make you feel superhuman, running on ketones won't prevent dangerous accidents if you decide running on the treadmill with your eyes closed is a good idea. Even if you're just walking, do not play along and momentarily close your eyes because I can guarantee there's at least one person in the row behind you that will point and laugh.

OK - so pretend close your eyes for a moment and let's talk about where you currently stand with keto. You've done the research. You've listened to the podcasts, and maybe you've read through a few keto books. You might even be a member of our courses. Perhaps you've already lost a few pounds on your journey.

You've done all of your keto due diligence, and you're ready to go into this low carb, high fat plan with a bang! You are ready for spectacular results, plus all of that extra energy you've heard so much about. You're even excited about a diet plan for the first time in a long time!

You no longer count calories since that's not what's important with keto.

With keto, you burn fat based on hormones, so calories mean absolutely nothing to you! Well, at least very little. You're a fat burner, so eat all the fat! In fact, calories, schmalories - you don't even bother looking at calories.

Your macros are set! You've got your protein dialed into a level where you'll eat enough to feel satisfied, but not too little where you feel shaky. Your fat is high enough to get you into ketosis, but not too high where you feel like a foi grased duck. You are ready to keto on!

Oh wait - before you keto, you almost forgot about the most important part - the carbs!

No one can succeed on a keto plan without first lowering carbs. And you - you're determined to become the next big keto success story, so you're going all in and lowering your carbs to 20!

That's right, you're not a cheater! You're ready to rock this keto thing the right way!

Are you motivated? And are you clear on your keto objectives?

If your eyes are still pretend closed, go ahead and open them. Now you have all of the info you need to follow a successful keto plan. Eat lots of fat, cut way back on carbs, and keto on!

And then ... then comes the fancy keto lingo like total carbs versus net carbs.

Just as you're settling into your keto groove, you decide to celebrate with with some bubbly - AKA, sparkling water, since you finally figured out *all* of the keto nuances. Or at least you thought you did.

But once you finally figured out what the heck a macro even is, now there are subsets of macros that you need to pay attention to.

What. The. Hell. Keto diet!

The Big Keto Debate

If you've followed a keto diet for some time, I know you've encountered the big debate: Net Carbs VS Total Carbs.

Not only have you encountered it, but you probably even formed an opinion as to which type of carb counter you are.

Let's face it - there are two different camps when it comes to counting carbs. You're either a total carb counter or you're a net carb counter. And unless you want to get into ruthless arguments on the keto message boards, you better pick a side and stand your ground. There are no gray areas permitted. You find your people and exit the opposing groups because in the land of keto, there can only be one way!

Wait, you don't actually believe that, do you?

I know I got you all riled up with the mere mention of those hostile message boards, but we're all different people made up of completely different body chemistries, hence we all have different needs.

I'm here to tell you that total carbs versus net carbs can become a gray area when it comes to keto, and those who insist there's only one way are hard headed bullies you need to avoid at all costs.

D'ya hear that, TracyandBrian?

In fact, if you're part of the keto support groups that insist you follow the keto rules *ONLY* as they see fit, run! Take all of the fat burning energy you have built up and run quickly out of those groups!

Even if you're not a fat burner yet, it only takes a few keystrokes to delete those groups filled with angry ketoers who obviously still aren't fueling their brains with enough fat, so get out now while you have your sanity.

They're not really support groups at all, and they will break you. If you disagree, members of those groups will badger you and scream at you how wrong you are! Even when you speak of methods that helped you lose more than 100 pounds, you're still wrong!

Group members will stalk you on Facebook until your 6'4, built like a linebacker, yet still a computer whiz husband, finds the stalker's home address just in case he needs to pay him a visit in person.

In the event you're not even on Facebook, and you have no clue what I'm talking about, let me start at the start and explain what net carbs versus total carbs even means.

Net Carbs Vs. Total Carbs Explained

Two people following a keto diet will look at this label and come up with a completely different carb count:

Nutrition Facts

Serving Size 1/2 Cup (69g)
Servings Per Container 4

Amount Per Serving

Calories 80   Calories from Fat 20

	% Daily Values*
Total Fat 2.5g	4%
Saturated Fat 1g	5%
Trans Fat 0g	
Cholesterol 45mg	15%
Sodium 160mg	7%
Total Carbohydrate 16g	5%
Dietary Fiber 3g	12%
Sugars 7g	
Sugar Alcohol 5g	
Protein 5g	10%

Vitamin A 2%	Vitamin C 0%
Calcium 10%	Iron 2%

*Percent Daily Values are based on a 2,000 calorie diet.

Some will look at this label and tell you this food only has 8 grams of carbs per serving, while others will look at your funny and let you know the label clearly states 16 grams.

So who's right, and who only learned common core math in school?

The total carbs in food is just as it sounds - the total amount of carbohydrates in a given food. These are the numbers listed on food labels next to Total Carbohydrate. They're typically the top number in bold print.

If you look a little further down the label, right below carbohydrates, you'll see a breakdown of the sources of carbs in food. The categories are typically sugar and fiber. Some labels might even show categories for sugar alcohols or other fibers. These labels may just show sugar alcohols, or they may even list out the types of sugar alcohols, like Erythritol or Maltitol. If you see a fancy word you're not familiar with that's hard to pronounce and ends with "ol," that's the name of a sugar alcohol.

If you're in the total carb camp, then you'll always want to look at that top number and count those carbs in your daily macros. If coming from the standard American diet, and you're still eating a considerable amount of processed food, even if it is labeled "low carb" or "keto friendly," then counting only total carbs can add up quickly.

Heck, even if you avoid these processed foods entirely and eat only whole foods like meat, eggs, cheese, nuts and veggies, 20 grams of carbs can still add up before you even make it through breakfast.

That's the reason some low carb guru coined the term 'net carbs.' If you see a packaged food that says it only has 2 net carbs per serving, but you look at the nutrition label and see the total carbs at 20 grams, I can see how this might confuse a lot of people who thought they finally had this keto thing down.

How the heck do the food manufacturers get 2 grams of carbs when the nutrition label clearly states 20 right there in bold print? It doesn't even make sense, you keto crazies! How has anyone ever lost a pound on this diet at all with so many confusing rules that change from keto expert to keto expert?

OK, I seemed to have gotten you all worked up again; at least in my head. Let's calm down and talk about how the food manufacturers got 2 grams of net carbs from a label that clearly states 20 grams of carbs.

The term net carbs refers to the carbs that your body processes and uses for energy - which are mostly carbs that come from starches and sugars. Many low carb gurus concur that some forms of carbohydrates, like fiber and sugar alcohols, don't count in the net carb equation because they pass through your digestion without breaking down. This means your body isn't utilizing them, so they don't think you need to count these carbs in your keto plan.

When you subtract out fibers from plant foods like broccoli or leafy greens, you can suddenly add a lot more veggies to your very low carb plan.

When you subtract out sugar alcohols, or even some of the fibers that don't naturally occur in processed foods, you can suddenly add a lot more keto candy bars to your plan!

In fact, some people may not even miss their old junk food ways since some of these manufactured keto foods are so delicious! Who needs a Reese's Peanut Butter Cup that will make you fat when you can just eat a 'keto friendly' peanut butter cup that claims it will help you burn through fat? Seems like an obvious swap to me.

Let's burn all the fat by eating keto Reese's!

If you raised your pitchfork high in the sky while screaming a collective, "Keto On!" you're definitely part of the net carb camp. If you're searching for some total carbers to lynch with your pitchforks, seriously, you need to get out of those keto Facebook groups because none of this is really all that serious.

I mean, sure, properly following a keto diet could be life saving for some people since too many processed carbs does contribute to poor health, which does contribute to killing people slowly. However, the people who are in that poor of health will most likely benefit from counting total carbs or net carbs, so let's all calm down a little and maybe pop a fat bomb.

Now the question becomes, when you pop that fat bomb, should you add the total carbs or the net carbs to your macro count for the day?

Even many of the foods you make at home with real ingredients will be different when it comes to total versus net carbs, especially fat bombs. They have ingredients like peanut butter and dark chocolate, which contain fiber. Many also add artificial sweeteners like Swerve to fat bombs, which claims 0 net carbs.

Now, I have to say 'claims' because when you look at a package of Swerve, it also shows 0 calories in a 1 teaspoon serving. Further review of the label shows 4 grams of carbs per teaspoon, which comes from Erythritol.

Wait a minute - it sure sounds like us low carbers have been bamboozled!

Even the novice calorie counter can tell you that there are 4 calories per each gram of carbohydrate in a food. If Swerve has 4 grams of carbs per teaspoon at 4 calories each, that's really 16 calories per teaspoon. So how the heck does the package claim 0 calories?

Ah, the epic force that is the food marketing department. Those evil geniuses have been sent here to confuse us all and keep us fat!

Food products like Swerve that contain 4 grams of carbs per teaspoon, but still claim 0 calories, can get away with that because this is considered a low-calorie food per serving. Regarding their claims of 0 net carbs, they're using that net carb theory I explained earlier.

The food marketing geniuses claim that sugar alcohols have zero impact on your low carb plan because they pass through your digestive system without breaking down. This means the products you use can have carbs shown on the nutrition label, yet still be labeled zero calories and zero net carbs.

Ah, the magic of marketing.

Before I talk about how I really feel when it comes to net carbs versus total carbs, let's explore this Swerve thing a little further. In real life there are 4 grams of Erythritol carbs per 1 teaspoon serving. When making fancy low carb desserts that taste eerily similar to our standard American favorites with ingredients like Swerve, most people will use at least a cup of this sweet stuff that tastes pretty close to sugar. Some with a severe sweet tooth might even use more.

Let's say you use 1 cup over a batch of fat bombs that makes 24. I just hit up Google and found out there are 48 teaspoons in a cup. Even though math isn't my strongest subject, I never learned common core, so I bet I can break this down:

- 48 teaspoons at 4 Erythritol carbs each is a total of 192 grams of carbs for the batch of fat bombs.
- We need to divide that by 24 fat bombs, so 192 grams of carbs divided by 24 fat bombs is 8 grams of carbs per fat bomb.
- This carb count doesn't include the carbs from other ingredients you use in the fat bombs, like nut butters or dark chocolate.

This means if you're determined not to cheat on your keto plan, and you limit yourself to 20 total carbs, you're done with carbs for the day after popping two fat bombs. No wonder people lose so much weight on keto - they're on a diet where they only get to eat two fat bombs, and then they have to starve themselves for the rest of the day. It's all making so much sense now!

Yeah, not so much. I've yet to meet a ketoer who eats two fat bombs each day and then lives and dies by a jar of coconut oil since there's not many other food sources out there that contain zero carbs.

If this is you, you are a magical person and I'd love to chat sometime. You also probably smell like coconuts.

The question here is how are so many ketoers adding fat bombs and desserts to their keto plan if foods these fat bombs contain somewhere around 8 grams of carbs per fat bomb?

That's the net carb approach. People who eat foods with sugar alcohols like this don't count those carbs because they've been told those carbs don't have any effect on their keto plan.

Many of these people also rely on convenience foods they find in the grocery store or online that cater to keto dieters because these foods market net carbs on the label.

The Net Carb Vs. Total Carb Winner

So who's right? The total carbers who strictly limit their plan to 20 total carbs each day, or the net carbers who can have seemingly unlimited carbs when they subtract out fiber and sugar alcohols?

They're both right!

Wow ... I just spent like 20 minutes explaining this whole net carb versus total carb thing only to confuse you even more with my conclusion.

I won't end this here, leaving you utterly lost and confused. This is a keto how-to book, so I want to teach you how to determine which approach you should choose for ultimate keto success.

Keep in mind, the following statement is my opinion. You'll hear varying views from different keto sources all over the ketosphere - but this opinion is how I've personally found the most success, and how I've seen others find long term success.
Also, it's not an opinion many ketoers will like. Please don't throw your artificially sweetened keto candy bars at me.

OK, I'll just say it - net carbs are for cheaters!

As I've been trying to teach my five year old who thinks cheating is something to be proud of, nobody likes cheaters! All of you net carbers are cheater, cheater, sneaky carb eaters.

Alright, I said it.

For those who've taken our Keto Decoded Courses, you've heard this. You already knew where I stood on the subject, so this revelation might not be all that shocking. For the rest of you, please sit down if you're feeling light headed. I understand I just completely rocked your low carb world as you know it.

OK, so I'm being a tad dramatic here. Drama just makes me laugh.

We all need a little more humor when it comes to keto because, man, there are just so many people who are far too serious and sciency about keto. They can speak their science, and I will speak my dramatic truth.

Now you might be thinking, "How can anyone possibly survive on a total of 20 carbs per day? Do they only eat meat topped with butter? Do they just drag a spoon through a big tub of coconut oil and eat as much as they can dig out? What else is there that doesn't make the carbs add up?"

This is why I stated earlier in this chapter that this whole net carb versus total carb debate can be a gray area; even for someone like me who thinks net carbs are for cheaters.

My Approach To Net Carbs Vs Total Carbs

When I first began low carb plans back in the day, I was fully entrenched in a net carb approach. I ate all the keto candy bars filled with all the sugar alcohols! Did I find success eating like this?

Mmmmm, kind of.

When I still ate a large amount of food as processed 'low carb friendly' foods because I didn't know how to cook, I did find some success on a low carb plan. At the time I was also fully entrenched in that diet mentality where I obsessed over counting calories, I obsessed over exercise, and I never felt great. Since the scale moved in the right direction, I thought eating tons of processed keto food was the right approach.

The problem is since I didn't feel great much of the time, and I wasn't eating real food that I also had the ability to digest, the success I did experience never lasted.

When I gave keto another go in 2015, I spent the prior year learning how to add more real food to my diet that was also lower in carbs. I lowered carbs per meal over time, so my body had time to get used to using fat and protein as fuel instead of using only carbs as my main fuel source.

It was also at this time I realized a lot of those foods marketed as 'keto or low carb' by proudly stating the net carbs on the front of the package weren't really helping my long term progress. I finally stopped buying into the marketing hype, and I focussed more on the real foods I still eat today.

This doesn't mean I'll never touch processed food ever for the rest of my life. This only means that over time I've cultivated a plan where the majority of the food I eat is real food that is naturally lower in carbs.

So long keto candy bars! Even though you're labeled as keto, you were still making me fat! You gave me a lot of gas too.

So what about the foods I make at home with higher quality ingredients, like sweetened fat bombs or keto desserts? Those still have net carbs, right?

I have two thoughts on this.

When I began in 2015, keto was still coming into its own as a popular diet for weight loss. This means there weren't keto dessert recipes everywhere you turned that were filled with sugar substitutes. I found a lot of my initial success eating low carb the old fashioned way. I focussed mostly on real foods that consisted of a lot of bacon, eggs, meats, fats and some veggies.

I actually didn't limit veggies at the time because they had too many carbs; I limited veggies because I didn't like them. My body had a full 34 years to learn how to live on processed junk that we've tricked into thinking is healthy. It took time and patience for me to learn to incorporate more veggies into my plan, and figure out that I needed the nutrients in these veggies to thrive. Veggies are also helpful in order to escape diet boredom when it comes to only eating meat topped with fat.

Even though I was technically a net carber at the beginning, I wasn't eating a whole lot of net carbs beyond natural fibers found in food. I found a lot of success like this.

Even as I found more options to add to my keto lifestyle, like peanut butter chocolate fat bombs, I still found success. At the time I was still in the bad habit of drinking artificially sweetened diet drinks, like Diet Coke, so I had a strong sweet tooth.

When I made fat bombs, I experimented with the different keto friendly sweeteners. Some of the sweeteners I used added carbs to my daily macro count, but I didn't include the sugar alcohol carbs I was told wouldn't count.

Guess what - I still found success! Many others who follow this net carb approach also find success.

Cool! Let's eat all the net carbs!

Well, I found success until I didn't. I was able to use a net carb approach up until I reached my ultimate goal weight of 135 pounds. I mostly used liquid Stevia as my favorite artificial sweetener because I figured out early on that sweeteners like Swerve resulted in digestive issues for me.

Anytime I ate a Swerve sweetened product, I ended up with severe gas pains. Instinctually I knew even though this sweetener was considered zero calories and low carb, it wasn't right for me. It also made me question the experts that say this has no effect on your digestive system since my digestive system reacted so poorly to Swerve.

I also subtracted out fiber carbs, so I was basically using a net carb approach to get to my ultimate goal. But it's still important to note I was eating mostly real foods. I didn't buy into the foods marketed as low carb or keto friendly. I never had success with those in my yo-yo dieting past, so it seems I finally learned my lesson when it comes to weight loss.

There are a few other important things to note that will help me slide nicely into my next point about net carbs versus total carbs.

While I'm no longer an over exerciser at the gym, I'm still an active person. I love to take long walks with my kids, and it feels like I'm constantly on my feet running around the house cleaning up or getting my kids snacks. I've also done a lot of work on my insulin resistance since I started low carb back in 2014.

The reason I want to point all of this out is even though I found success and made it to my goal even while counting net carbs, my total carbs were still likely in the range of 30-40 grams per day. Even though I followed the keto standard of 20 net carbs per day, my body was really finding success at 30-40 total carbs per day.

All of the work I did to improve insulin resistance, and all of the activity I get throughout the day, means for my keto plan I can really eat 40, or maybe even up to 50 total carbs each day to find weight loss success. In the end, that's the number I started to go by to find my carb threshold on a keto plan. I no longer wanted to do the math, so I began to view keto as a total carb diet.

I followed a low carb plan where I ate up to 50 grams of carbs per day to find weight loss success. For me to find success, those 50 grams have to be mostly real food, and not a lot of processed junk, aka, packaged foods bragging about net carbs on the package.

If you're not sure how to put keto meals together and you want a plan that's helped hundreds of challengers get big results, like losing 15, 20 even up to 25 lbs in only 21 days kind of big results, check out my Mix and Match Meal Plan. The plan contains nearly 60 keto friendly recipes that aren't chock full or sweeteners or other ingredients that lead to weight loss stalls. Plus, they're the same recipes I used to lose 100 pounds … and still use to easily maintain.

I also kicked in some bonuses to help you achieve amazing success with this easy and delicious meal plan.

But Everyone Else Is A Cheater, Cheater Sneaky Net Carb Eater!

So what about all of the low carbers out there that eat all of the sugar alcohols and still have success? Do sugar alcohols affect them?

It turns out, the keto community is very much divided when it comes to net carbs. Some still advise you not to count sugar alcohols, while others tell ketoers it's OK to remove them from daily totals.

Something else important to note when you're making this decision is a lot of people fall into the keto dessert trap. Many get really excited about keto because there are so many options available to them; especially options that are so close to their previous high carb favorites.

Unfortunately a lot of these people end up relying heavily on these sweetened keto foods, and their weight loss stalls, or sometimes even reverses direction. These ketoers don't understand what happened because they stuck to their 20 net carb goal.

If you follow a keto plan where you eat all the desserts, and you find tons of success counting only net carbs, I'm not here to ruin your day. I won't tell you that there's only one way and you need to stop this behavior immediately, or else suffer the consequences. You very well may be able to get away with that approach and still find success. In the famous words of Nene Leakes, you do you, boo.

For those following this approach, but you aren't getting the results you want, I think it's time to reign in the net carbs. Start approaching this diet from a total carb standpoint, especially if you're cheating on your keto diet with too many keto friendly processed foods.

You still may be able to eat some of these delicious treats, but I would advise saving them for a special occasion, or for a time when your carb cravings are high. Then, when you do indulge, it can feel like you're cheating on your keto plan when in reality you're probably not doing too much damage by eating these foods only on occasion.

That being said, if you approach keto from a total carb standpoint, that doesn't necessarily mean you need to limit your total carbs to only 20 grams each day.

Feel free to experiment to figure out if maybe 30 or 40 total carbs works for you. If you're not very active, or if your insulin resistance is strong, maybe you can only eat 20 total carbs per day. Take time to experiment with yourself, and come up with an individualized plan meant for you instead of just following the keto crowd.

What About the Veggies?

I've talked a lot during this chapter about those cheater, cheater sugar alcohol carb eaters, but what about the vegetables? Surely I'm not telling you to avoid nutrient dense vegetables, right?

Once again, this is another gray area in the keto world, so you'll have to figure this out for yourself. If you don't eat veggies because you're like I was and you just don't like them, just know that if you start eating veggies on a more regular basis, you actually will start to enjoy vegetables you never thought you would. I am living proof. In fact, you may even start to crave them, just as I do now.

No, I never believed that would be possible either. It really happens though, so if this is the only reason you don't eat more lower carb vegetables in your plan, start working them in over time. You can even try adding one new vegetable each week to see which ones you can tolerate. After a week or two of tolerating certain foods, you may notice you actually look forward to them because your body starts to realize the nutrients you get from them. It's like keto magic!

There are some keto dieters that can eat all the vegetables and still find success, while others can really only eat very limited vegetables if they want to lose weight. That's why so many keto dieters have moved onto a carnivore approach; they just don't do well eating vegetables or other carb sources, even when they count total carbs. Of course these people probably have work to do on their digestion, but tomayto, tomahto.

I personally would rather eat an occasional tomato, so I put in the work to improve digestion. Maybe some people are A-OK with only eating meat every single day for the rest of their lives, so they choose to let the digestion work slide.

No matter which category you fall into, I like to view veggie carbs as a gray area. What I mean by this is when I'm trying to lose weight, I still want to eat lots of veggies. I look at total carbs and see how high I can go in order to find success, while also incorporating adequate nutrient dense foods.

I personally find that if I focus on real food carbs with a lot of fiber, I can go higher and still find success. If you want to subtract out the fiber from these foods because it makes you feel better to see a lower number of carbs, go for it. If that helps you eat more fiber rich, nutrient dense foods, then do it! Subtract all the veggie fiber and go with that net carb approach.

Where I would suggest halting that net carb approach with fiber is when it comes to some of these weird non-naturally occurring fibers found in foods. You'll see them a lot in processed foods like cereals. Food manufacturers add them a lot of times to get the fiber count up in their foods so they seem healthier to consumers.

You might also see them in products marketed as low in net carbs, like low carb tortillas or breads. This is when I would stop the net carb madness. Sure, food manufacturers say that these carbs pass right through you, so you shouldn't count them in your total carbs; but these are the same food manufacturers that pushed low fat food products all throughout the 80's and 90's. These are the food manufacturers who destroyed so many people's health, and landed many of us shopping in the plus size section for years.

Never trust food manufacturers. Evil geniuses, every last one!

While I say counting net carbs is for cheaters, I do think people have a little bit of leeway when it comes to natural fiber that occurs in foods, like leafy green vegetables. If you eat a little over your carb goal for the day because you ate too many vegetables, that probably won't affect your progress.

I can't say this as a blanket statement for every single person out there, because that also wouldn't be true. Some people really can only tolerate very low total carbs to find success. As a general statement, most people will find great success on a keto plan when they subtract out veggie fibers.

When you start looking at other fibers from foods like cacao or peanut butter, these are also naturally occuring, but this one I'll leave up to you when it comes to subtracting the fiber out.

I'd personally leave it in so I didn't fill up on too many of these foods - at least until I found my keto groove and figured out what works for my body. Plus, if you're counting total carbs in foods like these instead of net, then the worst thing that will happen is you'll find out what your true carb tolerance is.

In case you're unsure what I mean by this, your true carb tolerance is how many actual carbs you can eat in a day to still find success. I think information like that is great to know and understand.

If you still heavily depend on keto processed foods sold in stores, you really should count the full carb counts in these products. Everyone will react differently to these, and you need to figure out where you land before you completely stall or reverse your progress. If you still want to eat them, at least you'll know why you may be stalled if or when it happens.

Also keep in mind a lot of these foods aren't real food. They are food-like products that have been developed in a lab to keep you coming back for more. Since they aren't real food, your body doesn't understand how to process them. This means they could be viewed as toxins by your body and stored in fat cells, even though they're labeled as low carb foods.

You should also consider that the sweetened versions of these foods likely contain undesirable sweeteners like aspartame or sucralose. Yes, some people still might find keto success eating foods with these chemicals, but I can tell you first hand that these chemicals are not doing great things for your health.

I ate artificially sweetened foods for decades. These were the same decades I struggled with yo-yoing weight. I also had a ton of health problems that have been associated with these products, like daily headaches.

Can I definitively say my headaches came from artificial sweeteners? Nope.

Did the headaches mostly stop once I cut artificial sweeteners from my diet? Yep.

Artificial sweeteners have also been associated with many other health conditions, so I suggest weaning yourself off of these sweeteners for good, and steer clear of them in the future. Stay tuned to future blogs or episodes of Chat the Fat, because there's so much more to the story when it comes to artificial sweeteners.

Chapter 9: Move Less, Eat More

Tale as old as time, song as old as rhyme, Nissa and the cardio beast.

Yep, just like our heroine Bell, exercise was a monstrous creature I loathed and avoided, until one day, against all odds, I fell in love with that cardio beast I once feared. I guess you can say exercise and I have a bit of a sordid love story.

Like lots of kids back in the elementary school days, I dreaded the week known as Presidential Fitness Testing week. I'm not sure if this was mandated in every school across the country, but it was a dreaded part of my childhood each May. In case you were never forced to partake, each year we had to show up in our gym uniforms and perform 5 fitness tests to the best of our ability.

These included partial curl ups, where you attempt a pull up with your arms facing in; right angle push ups, which are basically pullups, but also called a flexed arm hang for those of us too weak to complete an actual pull up; a v-sit, also called a sit and reach where you stretch out your legs into a V shape and stretch as far forward as you can; body mass index, where kids were informed of their body fat percentage using plastic calipers that squeezed their stomach rolls; and the most dreaded of all - the one-mile run.

I was a train wreck when it came to the Presidential Fitness Test. The v-sit was pretty much the only exercise I could complete without feeling extreme shame. My arms were far too weak to complete curl ups or pull ups, so I'd just hang on the bar until my time was up.

As far as the body mass index test, I absolutely hated having my stomach roll pinched in front of the entire class, because A. it's utterly embarrassing for a young girl to have her most problematic area pulled and pinched while her current crush waits his turn right behind her, and B. it f-ing hurt.

Then there's that one-mile run. Ugh. Thinking about that one-mile run still gives me PTSD.

Sure, these days I can run a mile in under 8 minutes, no problem. Some days I even look forward to getting a few miles in on the weekend. But back in my elementary through early high school days, I hated that one-mile run more than any other school task. I even hated it more than high school physics class, and believe me, that's a tough one to beat!

My high school physics teacher scared the bejeesus out of me! At the top of every class, Ms. Stein regaled us with stories about how she survived only on apple cores pulled from dumpsters as a kid in war torn Germany.

She paced the classroom floor during science experiments, scolding every last student. "You are not good enough for Champaign Urbana! None of you would make it at Champaign Urbana!" This was her gold standard of colleges. None of us could perform classroom experiments well enough to get into U of I, and we'd definitely never survive the cruel streets of Germany; or something like that.

My hand felt like it was at the breaking point of actually falling off my arm from extensive note taking during lectures, and I had actual nightmares about scrounging dumpsters for rotting fruit. But even as much as I dreaded that class, the one-mile run ran away with the most dreaded task each year.

Let me be completely honest - I never really had the ability to complete a one-mile run in elementary school, junior high or even through at least my sophomore year in high school. I always participated in more of a one-mile walk since I could never keep up with running past the first few steps. There was far too much huffing and puffing and feeling like I was going to keel over and die at any moment to keep going. I was always that girl who barely crossed the finish line before the end of gym class.

My extensive hatred of exercise changed once I became aware that I was a fat kid. I know that sounds harsh, but I stopped shopping in the juniors clothing section before I even entered junior high. The only clothes that fit were from the adult section, which as a young girl, it isn't so much fun wearing the same floral patterns as your grandmother.

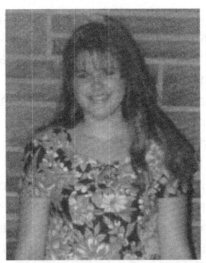

See - floral prints! Wearing grandma's finest to the 8th grade dance.

Once I became aware of my body, and I learned leaning down was all about expending more energy than you take in, exercise became my new best friend.

Earlier in this book I discussed the whole calories in versus calories out theory being a myth. While I still believe this to be absolutely true, it's a myth I fully believed and I fully perpetuated from a young age. It's a myth I followed before I even understood what calories were. Thanks again, high school physics teacher. You really taught me nothing beyond a general fear of women from Germany who were raised on rotten apple cores.

Exercise: The Full Story

To fully illustrate my views on exercise, allow me to share my exercise story with you. And I do mean the full story - the good, the bad, and the holy hell, how did I waste so much of my life following so much bad exercise advice?

Even though my life completely sucked every May during the Presidential Fitness Test, I still began exercising as an extracurricular activity at a young age. If I had to guess, I bet I was 12 or 13 years old. While I still fully hated running, I huffed and puffed my way through *Cable Fit Club* workouts, which mostly starred Tammy Lee Webb. Also, I realize I totally aged myself by name dropping Tammy Lee Webb.

Dating back to the days of watching step aerobics on cruise ships, while I clumsily attempted to follow along, cardio became life. I never allowed much time for stretching or weight training since most experts insisted exercise was all about the calorie burn.

I did attempt to follow *Body by Jake* a few times, and I also hung out with the older ladies of the PBS show *Body Electric* quite often, so I suppose I got in at least a little resistance training here and there. But I was really only interested in all the cardio, all the time. Fitness shows were scarce, so I took what I could get to ditch my childhood chub.

When I was old enough to score my first gym membership, it was like the best Christmas ever! Except Christmas in July since that's when I was finally of age. While some are excited to gain independence at 18, others get really excited to pedal nowhere as quickly as possible on a stationary bike.

My eyes lit up with glee during my first tour of Bally Total Fitness. Stationary bikes and stairmasters and steppers, oh my! No pushy sales person required since I only had to pay $19 per month to enjoy all of the cardio machines life had to offer. Sign me up for all of the gym memberships!

Thus began my almost twenty year love affair with cardio. I'm not even ashamed to admit, I was a cardio floozy. I switched my routine up, hopping from treadmill to stairmaster to elliptical, sometimes hitting all three machines in the same day. Thus began my decades-long habit of 60 minutes spent pedaling in place nearly every day.

When I wasn't at the gym sweating on the elliptical, I even took up running in my spare time. This same girl who wanted to curl up and die every May at just the mention of the Presidential Fitness Test began running of her own free will and volition. And I liked it!

While I previously kept most of my exercise and diet life a secret up to this point, I lived in a small town where everyone knew everyone, so everyone saw me huffing and puffing down the streets of Worth, Sony walkman in hand. Since the pounds consistently melted away, I was OK sharing my secret with the residents of The Friendly Village.

If you're brand new to my story, yes I grew up in a town referred to as the Friendly Village. The town's reputation did nothing for this girl who lives for snark. Perhaps the deprivation of adequate healthy fats to my brain turned me into a bit of a mean girl since at the same time I began this exercise routine, low fat was all the rage.

I typically ran the square mile that was Worth, IL, and then I'd hit up my favorite neighborhood spot, The Spaghetti Shop. Since running works up an appetite, why not order some low fat spaghetti, and wash it down with a pink lemonade? I worked at the shop, so my low fat carb up was even discounted.

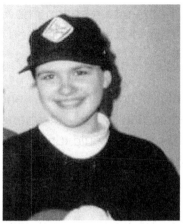

Fresh off the "run and then carb up with spaghetti and pink lemonade" diet.
'96

These were my humble yo-yo diet beginnings. I did all the cardio, and I ate all the low fat food to help me shed weight. And this plan actually worked.

You have to keep in mind, I was young and I went from eating a lot of fast food meals that were both high in fat and carbs, like a Burger King Whopper meal, to eating meals that were low in fat and high in carbs. While low carb isn't always the right plan for everyone, high carb plus high fat is pretty much a disaster for everyone.

My excessive cardio plan followed me throughout the majority of my life. Even as a busy college student who typically worked two jobs, plus had a full class schedule, I made sure to get cardio in every. single. day. Even days when I didn't feel well, cardio was my priority. I was that girl studying college books while blowing her nose on the elliptical.

Sounds healthy, eh?

At the time I was sure it took that level of commitment to reach my goal. Wait … did I happen to mention I never, ever hit a weight loss goal in the two decades I relied on cardio and CICO for weight loss?

My cardio obsession didn't stop there. After entering the corporate world, I tried to fit in a workout whenever I could. I joined a gym close to work so I could jump on the treadmill during lunch. I woke up at 4:30 am way too many mornings just to fit in an elliptical session. I skipped out on sleep, grabbed a can of low carb monster, and worked up a sweat before work. Other days I'd wake up early and grab a low carb SlimFast to drink on my drive to the gym so I had energy to workout.

When I became a mom, I'd be up half the night with my newborn, and then wake up an hour before my baby in order to get in some 'fat burning' cardio. Even after all of this, I sometimes lost weight, but it never stayed off for long, even with consistent cardio.

I did all of the right things to lose weight. I followed the advice of health professionals to a T. Now that my weight is stable and my health is excellent, I can look back and say I clearly had no clue what I was doing. Neither did they.

My Biggest Exercise Mistakes

All of the steps I took to get healthy and lose weight only promoted more inflammation, more stress to my body, and left me with less time for sleep. Everything I really should have been doing to help my body, I did the opposite.

Now stories are great, and hopefully you're learning from all of my mistakes over 20 plus years, but let me break down some of the biggest exercise mistakes I made for decades.

If you're still cruising along on your treadmill following in my footsteps, I'm letting you know you're getting nowhere fast. You can set that treadmill to top speed, but you'll still end up in the same exact place, huffing and puffing, thinking about how hungry that workout made you.

Without further adieu, let me break down the biggest exercise mistakes I made.

Mistake #1:

One of my biggest mistakes was over exercising when I was already overstressed with school and work. Excessive cardio added more stress to my overstressed body. Adding unnecessary stress to your body will never aid in weight loss. Stress spikes cortisol, which in turn makes it impossible for your body to switch to fat burning mode

Mistake #2:
Skipping over stretching and weight training so I could head straight to cardio was another huge mistake. Our bodies need to stretch for good mobility and health, and they need resistance training to stay strong and youthful. I avoided these necessities so I could get in an extra few minutes on machines that were holding back my results.

Mistake #3:

I hit up cardio machines or walked during my lunch hour when I worked in corporate offices. My basic routine to eat at my desk right before my workout to ensure I had energy to complete the cardio session.

Problem is, when I performed cardio right after eating, my body didn't burn stored fat; it burned the food I just ate. This routine led to even more hunger, and I always ended up reaching for a vending machine snack soon after my workout.

It was all very much a waste of time. Also, the only thing I really accomplished with this routine was continuing to inflame my already inflamed body with more cardio every single day since I overdid the cardio every single day.

Mistake #4:

Waking up at 4:30 am daily to get cardio in was a mistake I made for years. Not only is this going against my body's natural circadian rhythm, which is another way to stress your body, but I wasn't sleeping the 7-8 hours my body required.

Sleep is far more important to weight loss than more cardio. If you don't get adequate sleep, it's unlikely your body will let go of stored fat. Getting enough sleep will always trump fitting in another workout your body probably doesn't need.

Remember, a keto lifestyle is about balancing hormones, not about mastering a calories in versus calories out equation.

Mistake #5:

Waking up early for exercise after my baby kept me up most of the night goes along with what I just talked about. I'll keep telling you this until it really sinks in - our bodies need adequate sleep more than they need cardio. More stress and less sleep is a recipe for more weight gain; plain and simple.

Mistake #6:

I now realize grabbing a can of Monster or SlimFast are huge mistakes anytime of day, but particularly so around a workout.

Even though I chose the low carb versions, they're still filled with chemicals and junk sweeteners that spike insulin. That also doesn't take into account that eating moments before a cardio workout will only result in that food being burned, not stored body fat. Then you'll be hungry soon after and you'll want to eat again. You're basically spinning your wheels. And if you choose to spend your workout time on a stationary bike, then you're both literally and figuratively spinning your wheels.

Mistake #7:

Throughout most of this time I also restricted calories, sticking somewhere around 1200 calories per day. Since that's not nearly enough calories for my body to function, and I was never able to efficiently tap into fat stores since I never ate enough for my body to feel safe enough to do so, I required my body to search for its own energy for a strenuous workout. Since I starved myself of nutrients, my body was forced to break itself down to find more energy.

This is one way people wind up with chronic illnesses; and I definitely didn't feel well most of the time. When I first began testing chemistry, I always displayed a strong catabolic imbalance. This is a state where your body constantly breaks itself down. I didn't display the counter-balanced anabolic rebuilding phase of my day, pretty much ever.

This imbalance made me weak, caused daily headaches, and made it difficult for me to lose weight. The constant cardio I participated in since age 12 is a big part of what caused this catabolic state most of the time. If I didn't take time to correct this imbalance, it could have led to even more health problems down the road.

This is especially true with my current ketogenic and intermittent fasting lifestyle. Both of these lifestyle choices can push many into an even further catabolic state.

Exercise Truth

You're probably wondering why I waited until nearly the end of a weight loss book to talk about exercise. Every health guru out there hardly ever talks about changing your eating habits without also changing your exercise habits.

I'm here to drop some exercise truth. Please don't throw your dumbbells at me since this will go against pretty much everything you've been taught about exercise up to this point.

Exercise won't help you lose weight.

Well, at least not in the way it's been sold to you. Many professionals state a rigorous exercise routine is absolutely required to get you to your weight loss goal. In my extensive experience, this is untrue.

Most who parrot exercise being equally important to food choices, or better still, the foods your body is able to digest, still follow the calories in versus calories out myth.

Yes, I did just call out decades of expert touting as an absolute myth.

It's not the first time either! And I'll keep calling it out since we've all been brainwashed by this myth for far too long. This is *the myth* that took so much time for me to overcome, so I know exactly how you feel.

If hitting your goal weight was as simple as regulating the calories you take in versus the calories you expend, we'd all be at our goal weights by now because we've all unsuccessfully followed this approach for decades. Calories in versus calories out is right up there with a low fat diet being optimal for everyone. All that advice did was make us sick, unhealthy and fat.

A lot of people hear my exercise story and think, "Cool - I never liked exercise anyway, so I'm swapping my running shoes for a tub of coconut oil."

That's not what I'm saying here. The point I'm trying to make is while too much exercise, or exercising in all the wrong ways, can be a bad thing, exercise is still important for great overall health. It's important for us to remain active in order to stay strong and youthful. It's also important for improved mental health. Finally, moderate exercise can be a helpful tool in bringing insulin levels down, which in turn promotes weight loss. But, this is only true when done correctly.

If you spend hours upon hours every week on cardio equipment because you're sure that's what you need to do to lose weight, you could be hurting your progress. Too much exercise promotes inflammation, which will lead to weight gain. How many health pros tell you that side of the story?

If you're just starting out, and exercise isn't part of your daily regimen, please don't rush into a strenuous routine. Start off slowly. If exercise is too stressful, it won't help. Remember, more stress equals a cortisol spike, which could mean back to fat storing mode.

If exercise is a stress reliever for you, that's where you'll benefit. Relieving stress will put your body back into that fat burning zone.

After my first pregnancy I thought I needed to do all the cardio to cut through the baby weight. With changes to my digestion and diet, I lost somewhere between 80-90 pounds in between pregnancies. At the time, I still attributed this loss largely to early morning cardio sessions. There were many mornings I was sleep deprived, yet peddling away on my elliptical.

After my second pregnancy, we moved across the country with two small children. I no longer had time for constant exercise. I did my best to fit in fasted walks whenever I could, but there were more than a few weeks where packing and unpacking was the only exercise I could fit in. The gym quality elliptical I had for years was moved across the country basically to collect dust since I no longer had spare time.

Turns out, the 65 pounds I lost after my second pregnancy was a much smoother process than the 90 or so pounds I took off with my first. Beyond chasing kids around, and the walks I took for stress relief, I hardly exercised at all.

Looking back, I definitely would have benefited from more strength training types of exercises, but at that time in my life I didn't have time, and my priorities revolved around my kids. Getting enough sleep and keeping stress levels low became most important. Searching for time for formal exercise would have added unnecessary stress to my life.

Not having time to do more exercise did show me that the experts who tell you what you eat is most important in your health journey are correct. Many throw out different statistics. Some say what you eat is 80 percent, with exercise making up the other 20 percent of your results, while others say it's a 90/10 split with what you eat being 90 percent of results.

While I can't tell you which statistic is correct, I can tell you I lost 65 pounds and surpassed my original weight loss goal of 150 pounds with hardly anything I'd consider structured exercise at all.

My Exercise Truth

These days I do my best to make it to the gym - but only when it fits into my schedule, and mainly to complete resistance workouts to help out with posture and strength. If I do any cardio at all, I typically make time for 1-2 high intensity interval training workouts per week on the treadmill. I also walk with my kids often to stay active, but that's because I enjoy it. Since I enjoy it, this routine helps bring stress down, which helps bring insulin levels down. Staying active is important, and is much different than over exercising on cardio machines at intense levels.

With all of this exercise knowledge and decades of first hand experience of what not to do under my belt, there are still many chronic cardioers out there who love to argue. They tell me I'm wrong and that hours of cardio each day is exactly what they need in order to make it to their weight loss goals. If that's truly what you believe, cardio on!

I don't really love to debate over the merits of cardio. While I've actually come to love a good cardio session, and I occasionally use it as a reward after resistance training, I now understand while cardio might be great to help me feel good mentally when done in moderation, I no longer look at any cardio as a good calorie burn. I no longer abuse cardio so I can eat a few extra calories to help my undernourished body. With this keto lifestyle, I eat to satiation and exercise when I feel like it.

After what seems like a lifetime of over exercise, I reversed the advice of many health gurus out there. These days I actually eat more and exercise less for optimal health. For the first time in my life, I maintain a 100+ pound weight loss with ease instead of struggling through losing and regaining the same 50 pounds with endless exercise. This is what happens when you eat based on hormones, and when you eat foods your body is meant to thrive on.

Hopefully learning about my sordid exercise past helps you connect how exercise can play a role in your life. While I can't tell you which forms of exercise are right for your body, I can tell you to pick something you love, and be in it for the mental health and strength benefits exercise provides.

I can also tell you to learn how to exercise the right way. Quit wasting time with ill timed meals and all of the wrong routines.

Chapter 10: Supercharged Results, Real Fast

Intermittent fasting of some sort has been part of my success since the beginning, yet I rarely talk about the fasting methods I used to lose more than 100 pounds. I guess since I've taken the time to learn so much about keto and fasting, and since all of the information is readily available, I figure everyone else must be as big of a health geek as me. Everybody already knows all there is to know about fasting, right?

Anything you may have missed, I added to the Fasting Decoded Course, so we should be all caught up then.

Then I realized some people actually have lives beyond researching the latest health crazes. Some people get out into the world, eat at trendy restaurants, hang out with friends, and live their best lives instead of reading another diet book, so I'll take this chapter to expand on how I used intermittent fasting as a tool for faster success.

Some of the IF methods I used were only temporary, while others have become daily habits that stuck around long term because they've become part of my lifestyle. Some of these methods are more extreme than others, but I keep them in my weight loss toolkit for a rainy day.

Keep reading to learn all of my fasting habits. These are the same habits that landed me on the fifth page of a five page spread of *People Magazine's 100 Pounds Down Issue* in June 2018.

Sure, my fasting methods weren't mainstream enough to make the cover, and maybe it even seems they barely squeezed my story in, but the point is a national magazine helped make intermittent fasting at least a touch more mainstream. This final page of their feature article helped people realize *when you eat*, and not always what you eat, can play a big role with weight loss success.

While I didn't make it on the cover, and I wasn't flown to New York to be on *Good Morning America*, they did show my picture on shows like *Inside Edition* and *Extra!* These are the same shows I grew up watching, bag of potato chips in hand, while other kids were outside playing. These shows played at least some part in making me fat, and here I was with my picture displayed as the teaser story about women who lost 100 pounds.

Full circle moment.

Intermittent Fasting Truths

Those who don't know better look at intermittent fasting and say, "Well, of course you'll lose weight when you add fasting - you eat so much less when you skip meals!"

If you've been paying attention through this point of the book, you've surely noticed this isn't the way intermittent fasting works; at least it's not the way fasting works for me.

Maybe that's the way fasting works for some people. As I keep repeating, we're all different and we all need to follow a different path to optimal health. While there are some who will benefit from lower calories for weight loss long term, those aren't the same people who spent the previous twenty years in a constant cycle of restriction.

If those who've been overly restricting for far too long want to get off of the weight loss rollercoaster for good, they often need to provide their bodies with more nutrients it can utilize, not significantly less.

I'm looking at you Weight Watcher's addicts.

If you lost and then regained weight on this program several times in the past, why do you think this time will be a different story?

Yes, you and Oprah still get to eat bread. Bread!

Yes, you may lose weight again.

Yes, you will be hungry and feel deprived throughout the course of following this calorie restricted plan.

Yes, you will gain all of the weight back, plus more, once you can no longer sustain this lifestyle of nutrient deprivation.

If you insist on continuing this lifestyle, even after reading this book, please find someone that will shake you while screaming, "Jackie, Get ahold of yourself!"

OK, so your name's probably not Jackie. But calorie counting addicts, whether your name is Jackie or not, you need that kind of tough love in your life. And for those smug Jenny Craig followers or My Fitness Pal calorie counters thinking this doesn't apply to them, it's all the same poop, different day.

You thought I was about to say the "s" word, didn't you?

I do my best not to swear since my 5 year old is usually cuddled up next to me most mornings as I write. He hears and repeats everything, including some of the new words he's learning how to read.

In fact, just yesterday my husband arrived home from an exhausting business trip. The 5 year old begged him to glue legos together as soon as he walked through the door. Even though my husband was exhausted, he agreed since he knew the kid would keep begging until he wore him down.

Here's how their special family moment went:

Exhausted husband accidentally glues finger to lego and mumbles, "Shit!"
5 year olds asks, "Why did you just say shit?"
Mom laughs and shakes head at husband.
Exhausted husband snaps, "Don't say that word."
Exhausted husband accidentally glues finger to lego again and mumbles, "Fuck."
5 year old asks, "Why did you just say fuck?"
Mom shoots husband a glaring look.
Exhausted husband mumbles, "Don't say that word either."

Aren't these the special family moments we all crave?

You know by now I'm good for at least one tangent that has absolutely nothing to do with the current topic at hand. I hope that's as endearing as I mean it to be. After all, there's enough diet books out there that are all about sticking to the science, right?

I bring to you the science backed methods that worked for me, plus a dose of reality. I don't think you'd still be reading this far into the book if you didn't at least enjoy it a smidge.

Well, that's not completely true. Soon after releasing this book, some unruly keto-wannabe read until the end, and proclaimed she threw her book across the room out of frustration.

First, are we still buying actual paperback books? Is that a thing?

Second, she's not paying attention since if she had ketones in her life, she'd laugh along with the rest of you and realize she just got a whole lot of amazing information for less than the cost of a drink at Starbucks.

If I had much of this information twenty five years ago, I'd have nothing to write about since no one wants to read a health book by someone who never struggled in the first place.

Those one star reviews completely ruin my week, so now I only pay attention to those who leave five stars. Sometimes I even shout them out on my podcast!

Looking back to my two decade plus history of yo-yo diets, once I changed up my lifestyle with adding keto and intermittent fasting as everyday occurrences, I actually eat almost double compared to what I used to eat all of those years spent dieting.

To add insult to injury to those who believe fasting is all about suffering through a new form of calorie restriction, not only do I eat nearly double most days, but I also lost more than 100 pounds with this whole eat more, move less campaign. I currently maintain my lowest weight since before junior high by eating a whole lot of delicious food.

If you're thinking, "Cool! I'll just double up on my Lean Cuisines and potato chips because I want a piece of that weight loss pie."

Um, yeah; so it doesn't quite work like that. Also, today isn't Thanksgiving, so quit thinking about pie!

If now you're thinking, "Well thank you, Captain Obvious!" I learned in my short lived keto coaching career that what should be obvious to everyone isn't quite always the case. In fact, there are many assumptions I took for granted that I shouldn't have taken for granted at all.

Things like if you're making a recipe that calls for nuts, but you're deathly allergic to nuts, don't add the nuts. It should be obvious that you can remove a minor ingredient from a recipe that could kill you, right? Am I all alone in that assumption? Because a former coaching client, Rebecca, didn't quite understand that part. I'm only calling her out by name because I did everything I could to help her, and the girl was mean.

The good part is the people who this isn't obvious to probably don't even realize I'm talking about them, so it's not even like I'm insulting anyone. Even if they do realize it, these people shouldn't feel too bad. They're reading a book by the same girl who once upon a time thought pooping one time each week was completely normal. So there's that.

I've heard some of my favorite keto experts on other podcasts talk about adding fasting to their routine like it ain't no thang, especially when you're already in a fat burning state by following a ketogenic diet.

While that might be true for some people, going even 12 hours without food can be agonizing for others. Sure, just a few decades ago it was normal to go 12 hours or more without food, but we've since evolved into this culture who eats their 4th meal each night from Taco Bell.

If you learn nothing else from this book, please understand eating a 4th meal isn't a good idea, and food served through the Taco Bell drive thru may or may not be horse meat. I can neither confirm nor deny that statement. The sad part is, neither can Taco Bell.

How To Start Fasting Intermittently

If you're new to intermittent fasting, this is where I suggest starting: Stop eating after dinner, sleep for 8 hours, and then wait around an hour after waking up before you eat. When you follow this routine, you my friend, just completed a 12 hour fast.

In case visuals work better for you, here's what a basic 12 hour fast might look like:

- Finish dinner by 7 pm
- Go to bed by 10 pm
- Sleep 8 hours
- Wake up at 6 am
- Wait until 7 am to eat breakfast

Many are shocked to learn the time you spend sleeping counts towards your hours fasted. If you were to complete a 12 hour fast while you were awake, and then you sleep for another 8 hours, that would leave very little time to eat.

It's important to point out that a 12 hour fast is a very basic fast. If you decide to push your fast up to 16 hours, and then you sleep for 8 … while math was never my best subject, it sounds to me like you'd never have time to eat with that schedule. It sounds to me like you'd definitely lose a few pounds.

Let me be Captain Obvious all over again. Not eating because you're always fasting isn't a plan you want to follow if you, I don't know, want to do things like not die.

Ok, now that I continue on my path of insulting some of the very same people I'm hoping to help, let's move on.

Please note, I have mold brain. I know we haven't discussed it much during this book, but mold brain makes you mean. I'm trying to work on that, I swear.

I'm also still contemplating if I should write more about the subject in this book because, while this knowledge can help a great many people, it's a deep rabbit hole that once you go down, thousands of dollars and millions of frustrated tears later, there's no turning back.

So once I got the 12 hour fast thing down, I started adding even more time onto that schedule. Eventually most days I was able to fast for 14 hours straight without a whole lot of effort. I stopped eating after dinner, and since I typically ended dinner by 6 pm, I didn't eat again until the next day around 8 am.

Here's an example of what my 14 hour fast looked like:

- Finish dinner by 6 pm
- Go to bed by 10 pm
- Sleep 8 hours
- Wake up at 6 am
- Wait until at least 8 am to eat breakfast

Back when I was following 14 hour fasts, I was an early riser because I was a new mom that had a baby who refused to sleep for much of the night. Once he drifted off to dreamland for a few early morning hours, I took my sleep deprived self and snuck in a fasted workout.

While I don't ever recommend getting in cardio over more sleep, I do recommend a moderate fasted workout of some sort when you have time, as it really helps build up fat burning ketones. It can also help you fast even longer than you originally intended. I know it seems like it would be the opposite, and that working out in a fasted state would zap your energy, so I guess you'll just have to trust me on this one.

If you're not fat adapted, and you're rushing to the fasting part before your body is ready, you will hate me when you follow that advice. Since this is a book about keto and learning how to become fat adapted, I'm assuming you've got this part down by this point in the book.

Performing 12-14 hour fasts when you're not yet fat adapted can be ok for some people, but if you attempt to push fasts longer, especially while adding fasted workouts into the mix, you will hate life.

Quit doing things that make you hate life just to lose weight. If you learn to follow these plans the right way from the start, you can enjoy life, even while getting results!

Tony Montana said it best. "First you get the money, then you get the power, then you get the woman." Except with fasting, first you get the fat adaptation, then you get the extended fasts, then you get the supercharged results.

Sure, mine doesn't roll off the tongue quite the same way, but if you say it in the same mobster accent as Tony, that helps. For many, this is when extended intermittent fasts become easy!

When you become fat adapted, not when you talk like a fictional mobster.

Did you go back and reread that line in your best Tony Montana voice? I bet you did!

When I added intermittent fasting to my routine in 2014, there was no shortage of articles floating around that talked about the safety of intermittent fasting for women. Many of my most trusted resources said women should not fast longer than 14 hours for hormonal reasons. Since I didn't want to screw up my hormones anymore than I already had with more than twenty years of yo-yo diets, I listened.

If you can recall all the way back to chapter 3 when I talked about my first year in this low carb lifestyle, I had a lot of success by cutting carbs and fasting for 12-14 hours daily. If this is all you feel comfortable with for your current fitness level, keep at it.

There's no need to rush into more fasting or a ketogenic level of carbs if your physiology isn't having it. Rushing into plans you're not ready for creates stress. A stressed out body is a body that reverts to fat storing mode, no matter how hard you keto, or how much you force fasting.

Advanced Fasting Routines

If you're ready to push your fasting routine further, let me share a few more of the fasting patterns I followed that sped up my results. They also left me with a ton of energy, despite not eating for long periods of the day.

It's also important to note, fasting longer can lead to increased autophagy, which is a cellular cleansing that's great for improved health. I feel better adding this note since I don't feel like I'm only going on and on about the weight loss benefits of intermittent fasting.

Yes, I understand the weight loss aspect is probably the reason you're here. I want you to also understand that following a keto and intermittent fasting lifestyle has so many benefits beyond just weight loss. Soon enough, you may even be eating less carbs or fasting more in order to reap the health benefits, and weight loss may become an awesome side effect.

After I had my second baby in 2016, I got back to a keto plan as soon as I was ready.

I still have the picture I took the day I got back to my plan, which was six weeks after I had my newest bundle of joy ripped from my womb.

That's my dramatic way of saying he was another C-section baby. At 9 pounds, 14 ounces, I'm thankful he was another C-section baby. He came out large, and while he's only 3, he's at least the size of most 5 year olds because he loves his beet!

That's toddler speak for beef, which makes this keto mommy very happy.

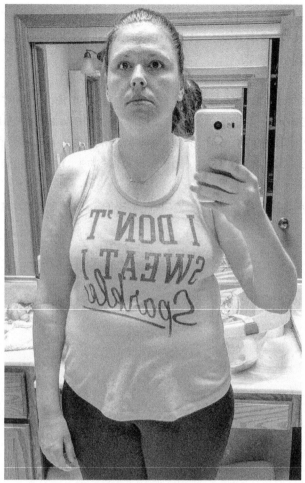

April 2016, six weeks postnatal - 195 lbs.

While I don't look very happy six weeks postnatal, I knew I'd be OK since I finally understood exactly what to do. I was also in far better health than after my first kid, so I felt like I was way ahead of the game.

Sure, I was back up to nearly 200 pounds, but as a new mom who was ready to keto it up, I felt like I'd be back to the goal weight I reached after my first pregnancy in no time. I had more than 45 pounds to go to reach that 150 pound milestone I celebrated pre-pregnancy.

I started back on a keto plan of only 20-30 carbs per day. I kept fat higher throughout pregnancy, so I was able to get back into ketosis pretty easily after my ten month break. Even though I still put on a significant amount of weight during pregnancy #2, I didn't go crazy eating all the carbs this time around.

Once I started keto again, I also added in 14 hour fasts to help speed up my progress. My body remembered this routine, even after a pregnancy break, so it wasn't too hard to get back into the swing of things.

At the risk of being scolded by all of the crunchy moms in the land, it's important to note I wasn't able to breastfeed. While that's another story for another day, I wanted to mention it here because if you're a woman who just had a baby, and you're still breastfeeding, adding intermittent fasting isn't a good idea until you're done.

Fasting while breastfeeding can mess with your milk supply. Making sure your baby is properly nourished is far more important than losing a few extra pounds. While intermittent fasting can lead to quicker weight loss, that quick fat loss will release the toxins you have in fat stores at a much quicker pace. These toxins will come out any way your body is able to expel them - including breast milk.

Eating keto while breastfeeding is a different story. I'm not a doctor, so I won't give any recommendations as to if you should eat keto while breastfeeding. It is interesting to note that babies are essentially born in a ketogenic state, and the breast milk that sustains them for the first 6 months of their life is made up of a lot of fat. Do your own research here, and be sure to check with your doctor.

After six months of following a keto plan this time around, I lost upwards of 25 pounds.

While that seems lower than most people would expect in a six month period, IT'S ABSOLUTELY NORMAL!

Please excuse my tone. I feel the need to yell at those who go into keto with unrealistic expectations, like expecting to drop 25 pounds each month. This isn't how weight loss works, and if you try to outwit this fact of life, you'll keep hopping from diet to diet until the day you die.

I already yelled at you; please don't make me point my finger too. You obsessive keto crazies know who you are - no angry finger pointing required.

Please understand that losing 25 pounds in six months is actually great progress. You should be very proud if you're able to hit such a milestone. Continuing at a steady pace like that until you make it to your goal, and then finding a maintenance plan that's appropriate for the lifestyle you want to live, that's what really counts.

I never thought I'd hear myself say this, but losing weight is the easy part. Finding a way to incorporate all of the habits you learn along the way into your permanent lifestyle is when the hard work begins.

Of course, if you follow along and do things the right way right from the start, the hard part just kind of falls into place naturally. Getting to and maintaining your goal weight becomes effortless.

Beyond the fact that losing 25 pounds in six months is completely normal, I had other considerations to take into account regarding how much effort I put towards getting back to my goal.

The second time around of getting back to goal, I had the stress of a new baby, some unwelcome family drama, oh, and did I mention we packed up our entire 3600 square foot house and moved across the country to Arizona?

No I didn't. Oh, and I also forgot to add that my husband started a brand new job the same exact day my second son was born.

Many say there are three big stressors in life: a new baby, a new home and a new job. I'd also like to add unwelcome family drama to that list, especially when your mom married the lead character from Dirty John.

We happened to experience all of these stressors at the exact same time. Taking what we talked about earlier into account, that a stressed out body is a body that lives in fat storing mode, I'd say losing 25 pounds over six months is a big frickin' deal.

Sure, at the time I would have loved to have lost more, but since I was dealing with a lot, I didn't stress myself anymore than life already was.

Right around the time we settled in Arizona, more information started coming out about intermittent fasting. Some of my favorite health authorities even changed their tune. Suddenly longer periods of fasting wasn't so dangerous for women after all. In fact, they now insisted at least some forms of extended fasting could help improve women's health.

As is typical for me, I went all Bill Nye the Science Guy on myself to see if this information was true. I still had another 25 pounds I wanted to shed, and like most dieters, I was ready to lose it yesterday.

That's when I began pushing 14 hour fasts a little longer to daily 16 hour fasts. It wasn't quite as easy as it sounds, but pushing my fasting times further in 20-30 minute increments every few days made it easier for me. There's no rush to hit that 16 hour mark tomorrow if your body isn't ready. Stressing your body out too much while adding a fasting routine can backfire, so take your time if you don't feel ready.

Remember, intermittent fasting is a lifestyle - something you add to your routine forever. While that task sounds daunting to the fasting newbie, adding intermittent fasting simplifies your life in so many ways and brings so many amazing health benefits. Once you train your body to adapt to your new schedule, you'll wonder how you ever lived eating more often than in an 8 hour window most days!

For me, a 16 hour fasting window meant skipping breakfast and waiting a little longer to eat an early lunch around 10 am. I did my best to keep busy in those few extra hours. Eventually waiting until after 10 to pop my first fat bomb, or drink my first BPC (bulletproof coffee), just became normal.

Here's what my 16 hour fasting routine looked like:

- Finish dinner by 6 pm
- Go to bed by 10 pm
- Sleep 8 hours
- Wake up at 6 am
- Wait until 10 am to eat breakfast

Keep in mind, I was definitely fat adapted by this point. Even with fat adaptation being part of the equation, sometimes you still need to take baby steps to get to that daily 16 hour mark. It's not always as simple as eat or don't eat.

If I'm describing you, take baby steps to get there if pushing fasts longer sounds difficult. You've likely trained your body to eat three meals and two snacks for most of your life. Suddenly following a new pattern of eating, like skipping an entire meal each day, isn't always as easy as snapping your fingers.

Once 16 hour daily fasts became as easy as snapping my fingers, I stepped it up and pushed some fasts a little longer. My goal was eventually to get to two days with full 24 hour fasts, while keeping to my 16 hour eating window on the other five days.

I want to reiterate here: when I talk about it now, this all sounds easy peasy, lemon squeezy. I can assure you that I didn't just wake up one day and fast for the next 24 hours. I was patient with my body and allowed myself appropriate time to adapt, both physically and mentally.

This means the first time I attempted a 24 hour fast, I probably stopped around the 18 hour mark. Perhaps on my next attempt I made it a little past 19 hours. I kept pushing each attempt a little further until I made it to my goal of a full 24 hour fast.

Once I worked my way up to two 24 hour fasts each week, this is what my fasting schedule looked like:

Sunday: Breakfast at 10 am, end dinner by 6 pm
Monday: Skip breakfast and lunch, eat dinner at 5:30 pm
Tuesday: Breakfast at 10 am, end dinner by 6 pm
Wednesday: Breakfast at 10 am, end dinner by 6 pm
Thursday: Breakfast at 10 am, end dinner by 6 pm
Friday: Skip breakfast and lunch, eat dinner at 5:30 pm
Saturday: Breakfast at 10 am, end dinner by 6 pm

There's no magic when it comes to breaking your fast at 10 am and ending dinner by 6 pm - that's just the schedule that happened to work for me. If your preferred eating schedule is different than mine, that's perfectly fine. The important part is to fast clean for somewhere around 16 hours most days, and work in at least two non-consecutive days each week to skip two meals in a row.

The meals you skip can be breakfast and lunch like me, or even lunch and dinner if you prefer a morning meal. If I didn't prefer to eat dinner with my family most days, I'd probably even skip dinner and breakfast on my 24 hour fasting days and settle for a late lunch since that's when I have the most hunger - but I like to have that meal with my family. Also, some days once I start eating, I don't want to stop … so skipping dinner might be harder than waiting until dinner to eat.

Working my way up to this fasting schedule was one of the best things I ever did to reach my goals. This was *the* schedule that helped me zip right past my goal of 150 and easily reach 135 lbs, a weight I hadn't seen since well before donning floral dresses in junior high. And believe me, once you get the hang of it, a fasting schedule like this is so much easier than it sounds.

Seriously - don't be afraid of fasting. I've worked with many of our Keto Decoded members who, even though they saw amazing success just by following keto, they waited far too long to add an easy intermittent fasting routine to their schedule because skipping meals can just seem so scary! Once some of these members implemented my easy intermittent fasting approach, their results skyrocketed, and they felt silly for ever fearing the fast in the first place. If you're still fearful like them, or you feel like you need even more info to get started on your fasting journey, I added my Fasting Fast Start Guide to the Mix and Match Meal Plan as a bonus!

And quite the bonus it is since following a proper intermittent fasting routine can save many upwards of $125 per month, while adding major convenience to their lives. Right now that extensive guide to start fasting the right way is only available with the meal plan … but with all of the value packed into the plan, it's worth snatching this deal up while you still can.

The guide walks you through every nook and cranny about how to implement an easy fasting routine into your keto lifestyle, including how to get started, tips to make extending your fast easier, the right way to break your fast for better results, and all of the frequently asked questions most new to intermittent fasting have. I truly wanted our members to have all of the best info when it comes to fasting since following fasting the wrong way can backfire big time!

If reaching a 24 hour fast a few days each week is one of your goals, keep working at it until you get there because it really is a magical moment. I still remember my first 24 hour fast. I kept myself busy that day with a stop at the chiropractor, and a trip to the grocery store for my eventual feast. I wanted to tell every Tom, Dick and Harry I ran into that I hadn't eaten in nearly 24 hours, and I still felt amazing!

Even though Tom, Dick and Harry are old school names, I'm sure there's plenty of them mulling about in Arizona during snow bird season. Even though I was ready to shout it from the rooftops, I kept this information to myself for two reasons:

Reason #1 - I'm pretty shy and rarely talk to strangers. I apparently only write embarrassing stories, like that time I took a mega dump, for strangers to read. But we're friends by now, right? We can talk poop stories for days!

Reason #2 - upon hearing I hadn't eaten for an entire 24 hours, most people would try to force food down my throat since the general public understands very little about a strategic eating window. We've all been trained by food marketing companies for so long that we need to constantly shove food down our throats, or we will die of malnutrition.

Guess what! Even at the time of writing this, it's 2 pm and I haven't eaten since dinner last night. So far I've written an entire chapter of this book, settled at least five arguments between my kids who've been fighting over an empty box all day, and I even got in a fasted OrangeTheory Fitness workout. I still feel great, and have no intention on eating until dinner. Fasting ketones are great for getting stuff done with extra brain power - even for those of us with moldy brains.

PS, a fasted OTF workout is another one of those advanced techniques. Kids, please don't try this at home; at least without more fasting knowledge.

Many Fasting Experts Are Wrong

This brings me back to the extensive research I've completed regarding intermittent fasting. Please understand that there is way more that goes into fasting than just not eating.

There's a right way and a wrong way to fast. If you follow the wrong way, fasting will be hhhhhhaaaaarrrrrddddd for you. I followed the wrong way because everyone on the keto and fasting message boards says things like, "You can have a tablespoon of cream in your coffee while fasting," or, "Of course you can have diet soda while fasting - there's no calories, duh!"

First of all, stop taking advice from people who end their sentences with duh. Their advice is stuck in the 80's, just like their choice of words. Second, while I like to give the message board participants a hard time, I've also read these tips in books written by fasting experts, or at least those I presumed to be fasting experts since they slapped their name on the cover of a book.

Fasting experts they are not because all of these tricks of the fasting trade make fasting hhhhhhaaaaaarrrrrddddd. Not only will following fasting tricks like these make fasting difficult, but in some cases, following these tips will make fasting far less effective. They may even lead to weight gain.

If you follow some of these 'expert tips' and fast ineffectively, you could be telling your body a famine has arrived and it needs to store more fat. This is when, even though you may be one of those fasters who eats far less calories, you could gain weight.

My husband is a perfect example. He was drinking coffee in the morning, and then had another coffee during the day. He didn't eat anything until dinner most days. The only calories he had up until dinner was a splash of cream with each cup of coffee.

If he's following the old school rule of calories in versus calories out, he should have crushed the scale each week, right? Except by not listening to the advice of his wife, or at least by only listening as well as my former client Rebecca, he actually gained weight while taking in fewer calories since he was now only eating one meal most days.

So about *only* needing to eat less food to lose weight ... doesn't seem quite so simple after all, eh?

That's my third "eh" of the book. All of my Canadian friends are proudly waving their maple leaf flags while singing, "Oh Canada, our home and native land."

I know I tend to make inappropriate jokes at times, so let me know Canadian friends if I'm taking this one too far. My kids are Arizonians, and they're only 3 and 5. I'm not fully prepared to go head to head with any angry hawckey moms, don't ya know.

Ok, focus back to fasting. Now that I expanded on some of the fasting things you shouldn't do, let's get back to some of the tricks that worked well for me.

Real Fasting Tips That Really Work

Here I was eating a ketogenic diet with around 20-30 carbs per day with plenty of delicious fat bombs to keep me in ketosis. Then I added 16 hour fasts most days of the week. I also took my kids for long walks to the park at least 3-4 days each week. Beyond that, I didn't participate in any organized exercise at the time. Once I was ready, I extended those 16 hour daily fasts 1-2 days each week to complete a full 24 hour fast.

For fasting newbees, a 24 hour fast is when you go a complete 24 hours in between eating. This doesn't mean you go an entire day without food. That type of pattern is typically referred to as a 36 hour fast.

A 36 hour fast is when you follow a pattern similar to eating dinner, skipping an entire day of food, and then resuming your eating schedule with breakfast on the third day.

What a 24 hour fast looks like for me is I'd stop eating after dinner, and then I wouldn't eat again until dinner the next day. There were typically 24 full hours in between meals, but I still had the chance to eat every day. Since I really like to eat, this was a great method for me. I was also sure to eat to satiation each time I had the opportunity to eat, both on fasting and feasting days.

Believe it or not, there are many nuances that fit into those 24 hours beyond just not eating. Aspects like how to start eating again, and how much you should eat can make or break your long term intermittent fasting success.

Eating too little or too much can wipe out all of your hard work. Since this chapter is getting long, and I'd probably just veer off into more unrelated tangents, I'll leave all of those nuances for my upcoming intermittent fasting book. I just started writing it, and it's hilarious (and more importantly, informative), if I do say so myself.

Of course, you can also check out our Fasting Decoded Course if you have the patience of a dieter who wants results now! We have detailed videos and PDFs that will walk you through every step of the way.

If you do take the Fasting Decoded leap, you'll notice the Keto Decoded course is a prerequisite. That's because we want you to learn how to fast the right way from the start. If you're not fat adapted through a ketogenic lifestyle, you could be stressing your body, which means you'll gain weight. Then you'll get mad at us because you paid for a weight loss course that made you gain weight.

Of course, we'll know the information you learned from our course didn't make you gain weight. We will fully understand that you're like Rebecca. We all know by now that Rebecca didn't comprehend weight loss coaching well.

Let's recall that Rebecca was deathly allergic to nuts. Rebecca thought she had to add nuts to a recipe because it was listed on the recipe, even though she was deathly allergic.

Rebecca almost died because she didn't use common sense. Please don't be like Rebecca.

If you don't follow through on being fat adapted before you attempt advanced fasting, you're not using the common sense instilled into you upon reading this book.

Thankfully 99.9% of the people reading this book are smart enough not to add ingredients to a recipe that will kill you just so you're following a recipe exactly how it's written. Staying alive is far more important than following an exact recipe. Did you hear that Rebecca?

Back to fasting and how I zipped right past my weight loss goal by combining intermittent fasting with a keto plan.

My original goal was to get back to the 150 pounds I hit after my first pregnancy. While I was able to diet down to this weight many times in my yo-yo past, I was never able to stay there for very long. I was also never able to make it to that weight without a whole lotta blood, sweat and tears.

OK, so I likely never bled to lose weight. Sweat and tears - yep, pretty much every damn day for more than twenty years.

When I set out on this lifestyle filled with delicious food that I was able to eat until I felt completely satiated, there was so much less sweat, and far fewer tears. When I turbocharged my weight loss by fasting the right way, not only did I hit my goal of 150 pounds, but I zipped right past it and dipped to 135.

Honestly, in all of my years of diet struggle, I never made it even close to the 130's. In fact, the last time I fell into that weight range was before I started shopping in the grandma section in junior high.

If you're reading this chapter with a smug smile attached to your face because you add cream to your coffee while fasting, or follow any of the other bad advice some other fasting experts provide, I once fell into your smug category as well.

I drank coffee with a splash of cream. I even added stevia, and I still lost weight. I used electrolytes that were artificially sweetened during my fasts too. Yep, still made it to my goal.

I followed a lot of the wrong advice out there, and I still saw success.

The difference is when I finally put proper fasting methods into place, that's not only when I saw the best results, but getting those results was no longer a struggle.

I too am one of the lucky ones who can still get results with a little bit of dirty fasting.

Now that I understand the difference with both results and how I feel, I'm no longer a dirty girl. Well, unless you've checked out my *Filthy Fast Plan*. I'm ok with playing in the mud with that type of fasting plan, but only if you follow it as it's laid out.

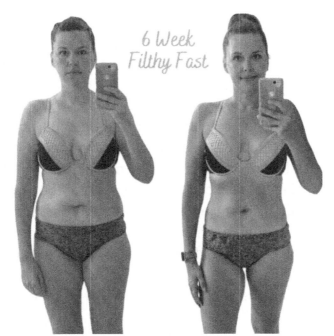

6 Week
Filthy Fast

Actual 6 week results after following my Filthy Fast Plan.

Conclusion

So perhaps this wasn't exactly like all of the other keto books you've read.

I used jokes in place of stuffy statistics, and personal stories in place of scientific studies. Please don't go giving me a 4 star review because I didn't get all sciency. I mean, I just referred to my lack of citing official scientific studies as not being "all sciency." Quoting official scientific studies performed by members of our society that hold PHD's wouldn't be appropriate coming from a girl who uses the word sciency.

Plus, some of the stories I shared with you my husband doesn't even know. He's too busy in his techy computer world to read this book, so I guess you might even know more about me than he does at this point. Bringing you to that kind of personal level deserves a full 5 stars!

PS … if you do happen to run into my husband after reading this book, ixnay on the poop sticks, deal? There are some things he doesn't need to know. Me telling the keto world that my husband uses mini plywood that resembles long chopsticks to break apart his poops are one of them.

I suppose if he did find out, it's not like our marriage would end. He maybe even deserves such tidbits of info leaking out as payback from some of the things he puts out into the universe. Like everytime I use the restroom, even just to pee or wash my hands, he says, "Mommy has to take a dump."

We all know how kids repeat everything they hear. Just the other day my 3 year old knocked on the bathroom door and with a concerned tone he asked, "Mommy, you take dump?"

Here I am, four paragraphs into my official conclusion and I'm telling you about how my 3 year old asks mommy if she's taking a dump. Seriously, I don't even know what's wrong with me and my big old tangenty brain. Must be the mold!

Oh, right … and that's something else I teased and left as a loose end. I actually went into this conclusion full well knowing that I never got to the mold story. Since it's estimated 1 in every 5 people are sensitive to toxic mold, and I fell face first into that 1 out of the 5, it's something I unfortunately know too much about.

The thing is, I'm only midway through my overcoming toxic mold story, so I figure that's a story best saved for another day, or at least until my brain is healed enough to give the full story. Plus, that gives me purpose to write another book filled with unrelated tangents. Win-win!

With this book, I didn't break down which exact keto macros *you* should follow, or which are the best fats for *you* to eat. I didn't provide a breakthrough meal plan or tell you how many calories to eat for ultimate success.

While I touched on some of that on a very surface level throughout the book, things like that are mostly individual. In fact, if I asked you right now, "What's the biggest lesson you learned throughout this book?" what would your answer be?

If you robotically recite, "If you have fat to burn on your body, you don't need to add fat to your meals," then please slap yourself in the head since I'm not there to do it for you.

Also, you need a do over on pretty much this entire book. Pay special attention to the Rebecca stories. Rebecca didn't listen very well. Neither did you if you still believe this keto myth that obviously makes me very angry.

What you should have been jumping around, hand in the air, eagerly awaiting to shout to the class is, "We are all individual."

What works for me might not work for you. That means if I were to give you the exact macros of what *you* should eat for keto to be a successful plan for you, I'd be a big fat liar. I'd just be throwing random numbers out, and hoping they stick.

That's pretty much what the entire diet industry is, right? 'Experts' who throw out tricks that work for maybe 50% of the people who follow them, while those tricks make the other 50% even fatter than when they began.

If that leaves you confused and feeling utterly hopeless, "Stahp it Rahn."

Sitting around feeling sorry for yourself with a tub of Ben & Jerry's isn't the answer. I can at least get that specific. I've put plenty of information in this book to help you find success along your merry keto way! I've linked the H-E double hockey sticks out of this book, and filled it with resources you can use to find the answers you need; some paid, but many free.

I'd like to say I'm sorry if all of the links offended you, but I'm really not. I've been at this keto game for more than six years, and I've been sharing my knowledge to help others change their lives for more than three. That's a whole lotta knowledge to share … and it's worked since I've helped so many others (both clients and book readers) hit major weight loss goals they struggled with hardcore prior to coming across my work.

Just in the last week alone, I've come across two people I've never talked to previously, nor did I know these people existed, and they both lost more than 100 pounds since first finding one of my books. They took what they learned with all of these 'offensive links' and took action, changing their lives forever in the most amazing ways.

And while you can get some pretty amazing results just by following what you've learned in this book, why not get even better results by having *all of the information* available at your fingertips? Literally, click the links and you have every bit of info I used to reach my weight loss goal for the first time ever. And if the links really do offend you, pretend close your eyes when you come across one.

Just when I got Carly Simon out of my head, she's making her way right back in! But at the risk of thinking this song is about me, it's important to note that I didn't just stumble upon keto, read one book and then poof - lifelong success.

I read that first book, and then I kept learning. I kept digging for the answers I needed in order to improve upon what I already learned and to continue my weight loss momentum.

(Someone was offended by my link dropping in a book review, which is why I stopped reading reviews any less than 5 stars. You can see how much those negative reviews infiltrate me to the core, and then I just won't let it go.)

In case you missed any of the previous *offensive* links I dropped, you can comb through previous blogs, my other books, my growing list of videos on YouTube, our Chat the Fat podcast or even the Keto Decoded Courses. We also run free workshops where you can learn how to overcome common keto roadblocks, and we have a free Keto Kickstart Course, which details the simple steps I used to get started on my 100 pound weight loss journey.

If you're up for a little friendly competition, plus the chance to win $500, I run a new Keto Challenge every quarter! And if you don't want to wait for a new challenge to begin, you can get all of the same info challengers use to lose up to 25 lbs in only 21 days with the Keto Quick Start Course.

So. Many. Opportunities. So. Much. Information.

In order to find lasting success on your keto plan, you have to find the right experts to follow, and stick with them. Following every keto Tom, Dick and Harry expert out there will lead to confusion because you won't know which keto advice is right for you. Even in the segmented world of keto, views and advice vary greatly.

I'd personally probably follow one of the keto experts who struggled for decades in the diet industry, only to figure out the path to individualizing a plan for her, which ultimately led to a whole lot of lasting success.

Following someone like that who's been in the trenches and was able to dig her way out over someone who's only looking at the studies to lead people down their keto path … meh, sometimes those studies aren't so trustworthy.

With many weight loss studies, oftentimes only the points that benefit the author's theories are used, while the other not so benefity points are swept under the carpet.

Real experience though … to me, real experience trumps bought studies anyday. And I was talking about following my continued work, in case that part wasn't obvious.

Perhaps you noticed some of this book wasn't even about keto at all. I spent two full chapters talking all about low carb, and then an additional three chapters hashing out digestion specific topics.

I personally needed to follow low carb to allow my body adequate time to adjust, just as much as I needed to improve aspects of digestion before I could find any level of lasting success on keto.

If you're not as badly broken as I was, I hope you read those chapters for the therapy sessions, and then moved onto the juicy nuggets of helpful keto info.

Now if that really is you, I hope you take those chapters seriously. Sticking your fingers in your ears while reading a book doesn't work well, remember? If you attempt keto and find bits and pieces of success without improving some of these digestive issues we talked about, you probably won't have lasting success.

I don't want you to follow a plan that eventually you'll give up on, or a plan will give up on you. Then you're back to square one.

Been there, done that - no thank you to that yo-yo lifestyle!

If there are points made in this book that you don't agree with, please don't stalk me on social media to berate me into your point of view.

I'm not about that life, and a simple unfollow will do. I blocked all of the TracyandBrian's of the world because I just don't care enough to argue with them. I like to fill my keto life with positivity, and the understanding that different things work for different people. There is no one way.

If you find something you don't agree with, move past that section and find different tips that will help you. Just know that these experiences are my own. Everything I wrote about in this book helped me lose more than 100 pounds, and I've kept that hundred pounds off for three full years now. I've since helped hundreds of others make it to their goals with these same tactics.

If you look around at statistics, that's not an easy task. If these viewpoints worked so well for me, surely they can help others out there as well, and that's really my only agenda.

It's estimated that for those who lose a lot of weight, roughly 95% of those people gain back all of that weight. Some even gain a little extra.

I fell into that 95% statistic for more than twenty years. It's not by coincidence that I've finally been resting comfortably with the other five percenters. I put in the work this time, and I did what needed to be done for lasting success. In this book I provide you the exact steps I took to get to the other side.

The awesome part is, since I put in the work up front, the side of keeping the weight off is so much easier. I basically live my life and I maintain with ease. Beyond eating delicious keto food combined with a few workouts each week to get stronger, it's really no work at all. I actually wonder how many of those other five percenters feel the same way. Just because they're keeping the weight off, it doesn't mean their life is easy like mine.

I don't want to be a lonely five percenter. Take this information I delivered and come join me! If you get stuck, then literally, come join me.

I set up an Eating Fat is the New Skinny Support Group on Facebook where you can ask all of your questions. If you need more help beyond just a few questions, we have entire courses set up to help you find your path to success. With either option, you're in great hands.

Before I leave you and officially conclude this book, I set up a free roadmap to how I found success. This might be helpful in case you forgot to take notes and you don't want to read this entire book from scratch. If you want to get my free weight loss roadmap, check out eatingfatisthenewskinny.com/roadmap.

So that's about all I have to say about how to succeed on keto without really trying.

Goodbyes are kind of awkward, right? Especially for stay-at-home moms who don't get out much since their kids hold them hostage with *Mickey Mouse Clubhouse* reruns.

Do we virtually hug? Maybe a kiss on the cheek?

Since I usually have coconut oil on my lips, I guess we should skip the kisses. That meme going around that says, "I have 99 problems and coconut oil solved 86 of them," is truth!

I'll just wish you lots of healthy fat love, and hopefully we'll see each other soon in one of the support groups, or maybe my next book. I've left you plenty of links throughout this book to find me, so let's break bread … or I guess in our case, bacon.

More About Nissa Graun:

Nissa Graun is the author of _My Big Fat Life Transformation_ and _The Lazy Keto Gourmet_. She is the co-creator of the Keto Decoded Courses, which includes the Keto Decoded, Fasting Decoded, The Fat Loss Course, Keto Cooking Decoded, Low Carb Cooking Decoded and Virtual Coaching courses. These courses are helping new people find their path to low carb, high fat success every day.

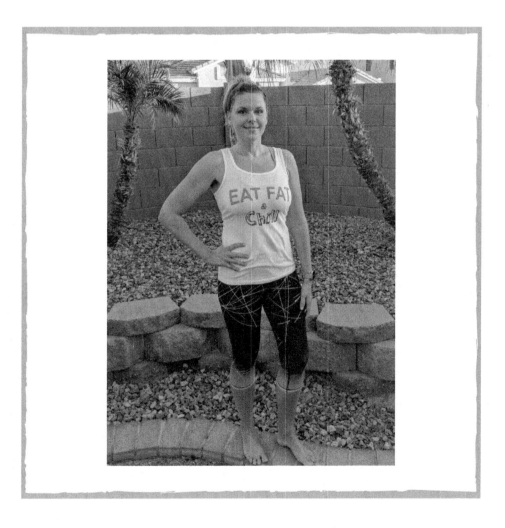

Nissa's weight loss transformation story has been featured in *People Magazine*, *People TV*, news stations throughout the country and health & wellness podcasts. Go to eatingfatisthenewskinny.com to learn more.

Join my Facebook group   Follow me on Instagram   Follow Me on Facebook

My Story:

I followed mainstream diet advice for more than 25 years. I was constantly sick, tired and miserable for the majority of those two plus decades.

Sometimes I lost weight, but it was always a difficult process and I routinely gained everything back within a year. Several chronic illnesses also plagued me for decades.

After hitting an all time high of 245 pounds after the birth of my first son, I felt completely helpless. All of my previous weight loss methods were useless. I was fat, sick, and miserable while still wearing maternity clothes more than a year after pregnancy.

I came across new information that changed my life. I learned how to use natural supplements and nutrition to take off the weight (for good), while also improving the health issues that I suffered with for longer than I can remember.

I set out with intentions of dropping weight that wouldn't budge via any other method, and unintentionally corrected health problems that afflicted me for decades.

Now that my health is thriving, I help others get off the yo-yo diet rollercoaster and drastically improve their health with my podcast, books, personal coaching and courses.

Resources:

Get My Free Guide:
http://www.eatingfatisthenewskinny.com/freeguide

Learn More:

Website: http://www.eatingfatisthenewskinny.com
(blogs, recipes, videos & more)

Digestion Course:
http://www.eatingfatisthenewskinny.com/fixme

Chat the Fat podcast: http://www.chatthefat.com
(find on your favorite podcast app!)

Books: http://www.eatingfatisthenewskinny.com/books

Supplements Mentioned:
http://www.eatingfatisthenewskinny.com/fixme

Keto Decoded Membership:
http://www.eatingfatisthenewskinny.com/kdmembership

Keto Quick Start Course:
http://www.eatingfatisthenewskinny.com/quickstart

Mix and Match Meal Plan:
http://www.eatingfatisthenewskinny.com/mealplan

Free Troubleshooting Keto Workshop:
http://www.chatthefat.com/workshop

Be social - let's connect!

Facebook: http://www.facebook.com/eatingfatisthenewskinny

Join my Facebook Group:
http://www.facebook.com/groups/eatingfatisthenewskinny

Instagram:
http://www.instagram.com/eatingfatisthenewskinny

YouTube: bit.ly/eatingfatisthenewskinny

Made in the USA
Middletown, DE
27 August 2023

37450010R00149